K. A. Lehmann D. Zech (Eds.)

Transdermal Fentanyl

A New Approach to Prolonged Pain Control

With 57 Figures and 37 Tables

Springer-Verlag
Berlin Heidelberg New York
London Paris Tokyo
Hong Kong Barcelona
Budapest

Prof. Dr. Dr. Klaus A. Lehmann
Dr. Detlev Zech

Institut für Anaesthesiologie und
Operative Intensivmedizin
Universität Köln
Joseph-Stelzmann-Str. 9
D-5000 Köln 41

ISBN-13: 978-3-540-54440-1 e-ISBN-13: 978-3-642-76872-9
DOI: 10.1007/978-3-642-76872-9

Library of Congress Cataloging-in-Publication Data
Transdermal fentanyl / K. A. Lehmann, D. Zech (eds.).
p. cm.
Results of a workshop held in Cologne, Federal Republic of Germany, Sept. 27–28, 1990.
Includes index.

1. Fentanyl - Congresses. 2. Transdermal medication - Congresses.
I. Lehmann, K. A. (Klaus A.) II. Zech, D.
[DNLM: 1. Administration, Cutaneous - congresses. 2. Fentanyl - administration & dosage - congresses. 3. Fentanyl - therapeutic use - congresses. 4. Pain - drug therapy - congresses. QV 89 T772 1990]
RD86.F45T73 1991
615'.783--dc20
DNLM/DLC
for Library of Congress 91-5144
CIP

27/3140-543210 – Gedruckt auf säurefreiem Papier

Preface

Pain is a serious clinical problem requiring considerable effort by physicians and the nursing staff. Although many methods of effective pain management are available, in daily practice the clinical outcome leaves much to be desired.

The medical community should not simply wait for "better" or more "modern" techniques to be developed but should play an active role in solving these problems. Gradually new, really promising strategies are being introduced. Transdermal administration of a variety of drugs, including cardiovascular drugs, antiemetics and hormones, has become a well-established modality. Experience with opiates administered transdermally goes back several years; most recently the transdermal therapeutic system (TTS) fentanyl was approved by the United States Food and Drug Administration.

I am pleased to present the results of a comprehensive international workshop entitled "Transdermal Fentanyl," held in Cologne, Federal Republic of Germany from September 27–28, 1990. Its purpose was to facilitate critical evaluation of theoretical and clinical studies on the new, noninvasive application of fentanyl, and to provide an opportunity for an exchange of ideas concerning its value for pain management, anesthesiology, and future investigations in this field.

The reader will find that the experts appreciated the value of transdermal analgesia but also warned against uncritical optimism. Experience to date has shown that TTS fentanyl can be a valuable tool in the clinician's armamentarium against pain. It should, however, be kept in mind that it represents a new application mode and not a new drug, and that sustained, noninvasive application requires careful diagnosis and good general standards of pain management.

The future will show which patients profit best from TTS fentanyl. May this book help the physician to identify such patients and offer encouragement to provide other effective methods of pain management to those who are possibly better off with conventional techniques.

I gratefully acknowledge the help of all the speakers and discussants at the workshop and the generous support of the meeting, provided by STADA AG Arzneimittel, which greatly facilitated speedy publication of the proceedings.

Cologne, Spring 1991 Klaus A. LEHMANN

Contents

Contributors

VON BORMANN, BENNO
Abteilung Anaesthesiologie und Operative Intensivmedizin,
St. Johannes-Hospital, An der Abtei 7–11, 4100 Duisburg 11,
Federal Republic of Germany

CHAPMAN, C. RICHARD
Departments of Anesthesiology and Psychiatry and Behavioral Sciences,
University of Washington, Seattle, WA 98195, USA

CHRIST, RAINER
E. Merck, Frankfurter Str. 250, 6100 Darmstadt,
Federal Republic of Germany

DUBOIS, MICHEL Y.
Department of Anesthesiology, Georgetown University, Medical Center,
3800 Reservoir Road NW, Washington DC 20007, USA

EBERLEIN, H. J.
Institut für Anaesthesiologie und Operative Intensivmedizin, FU Berlin,
Klinikum Charlottenburg, Spandauer Damm 130, 1000 Berlin 19,
Federal Republic of Germany

EINNOLF, CHRISTIANE
Institut für Anaesthesiologie und Operative Intensivmedizin, FU Berlin,
Klinikum Charlottenburg, Spandauer Damm 130, 1000 Berlin 19,
Federal Republic of Germany

GOURLAY, GEOFFREY K.
Pain Management Unit, Flinders Medical Centre, Bedford Park,
Adelaide SA 5042, Australia

GROND, STEFAN
Institut für Anaesthesiologie und Operative Intensivmedizin,
Universität Köln, Joseph-Stelzmann-Straße 9, 5000 Köln 41,
Federal Republic of Germany

GUPTA, SUNEEL
Alza Corporation, 950 Page Mill Road, Palo Alto, CA 94303-0802, USA

HWANG, STEPHEN S.
Alza Corporation, 950 Page Mill Road, Palo Alto, CA 94303-0802, USA

KNOWLES, MARK
Alza Corporation, 950 Page Mill Road, Palo Alto, CA 94303-0802, USA

LATASCH, LEO
Abteilung für Anaesthesie und Wiederbelebung, Universitätsklinik Frankfurt am Main, Theodor-Stern-Kai 7, 6000 Frankfurt am Main, Federal Republic of Germany

LEHMANN, KLAUS A.
Institut für Anaesthesiologie und Operative Intensivmedizin, Universität Köln, Joseph-Stelzmann-Straße 9, 5000 Köln 41, Federal Republic of Germany

LYNCH, JOHN
Institut für Anaesthesiologie und Operative Intensivmedizin, Universität Köln, Joseph-Stelzmann-Straße 9, 5000 Köln 41, Federal Republic of Germany

MATHER, LAURENCE E.
Department of Anaesthesia and Pain Management, The University of Sydney, Royal North Shore Hospital, St. Leonards, NSW 2065, Australia

MOINPOUR, CAROL M.
Pain and Toxicity Research Program, Fred Hutchinson Cancer Research Center, 1124 Columbia Street, Seattle, WA 98104, USA

NICHOLS, KIRSTIN C.
Alza Corporation, 950 Page Mill Road, Palo Alto, CA 94303-0802, USA

NIMMO, WALTER S.
Inveresk Clinical Research Ltd, Research Park Riccarton, Edinburgh EII 14 4AP, United Kingdom

PAYNE, RICHARD
Department of Neurology, University of Cincinnati Medical Center, 231 Bethesda Avenue, Cincinnati, Ohio 45267, USA

SOUTHAM, MARY A.
Alza Corporation, 950 Page Mill Road, Palo Alto, CA 94303-0802, USA

STREISAND, JAMES B.
Department of Anesthesiology, University of Utah School of Medicine, 50 North Medical Drive, Salt Lake City UT 84132, USA

STRUMPF, MICHAEL
Institut für Anaesthesiologie, Bergmannsheil, Universität Bochum, Gilsingstraße 14, 4630 Bochum 1, Federal Republic of Germany

TIGERSTEDT, IRMA
Department of Anaesthesia, Helsinki University Central Hospital, Haartmaninkatu 4, SF-00290 Helsinki, Finland

ZECH, DETLEV
Institut für Anaesthesiologie und Operative Intensivmedizin, Universität Köln, Joseph-Stelzmann-Straße 9, 5000 Köln 41, Federal Republic of Germany

ZENZ, MICHAEL
Institut für Anaesthesiologie, Bergmannsheil, Universität Bochum, Gilsingstraße 14, 4630 Bochum 1, Federal Republic of Germany

Part I. Transdermal Therapeutic Systems – An Introduction

Transdermal Permeation: Physiological and Physicochemical Aspects

S. S. HWANG, K. C. NICHOLS, and M. SOUTHAM

Introduction

Prior to the introduction of transdermal delivery systems, topical delivery of drugs was achieved by application of ointments or creams to intact skin. When the goal was systemic therapy (e.g., nitroglycerin and estradiol ointments), reproducible dosing was extremely difficult to achieve because of the difficulty in applying uniform amounts of ointment over a fixed area of skin. In addition, differences in the rate and extent of drug absorption could occur because of differences among individuals in the intrinsic permeability of skin. The skin site [8, 2] and skin metabolism [9] also contributed to the variability of transdermal drug delivery.

The use of skin as a reproducible route to deliver drugs into the bloodstream requires knowledge of the barrier properties of the skin so that the system can be designed to have more control over the rate of drug delivery than the most impermeable skin. The potency and physicochemical properties and the absence of irritation or sensitization determine the suitability of a drug for delivery through this route.

We will discuss the development of the rate-controlled Transdermal Therapeutic System (TTS) for systemic delivery of fentanyl. TTS (fentanyl) provides a convenient regimen for the use of a drug previously limited by a short duration of action as well as a noninvasive parenteral route for a drug that is unsuitable for oral administration.

Effect of Physiological Properties of Skin

Anatomy

The skin is composed of three layers (Fig. 1). The stratum corneum forms the outermost layer and consists of 10 to 20 layers of flattened, closely-packed, keratinized cells without nuclei. The epidermis, 50–100 μm thick, has rapidly dividing basal cells that flatten as they move into the stratum corneum to replace cells that are constantly sloughed from the surface of the stratum corneum. The dermis, 2000–3000 μm thick, is a matrix of various cells including collagen, elastin and reticulum [6]. Skin appendages include hair

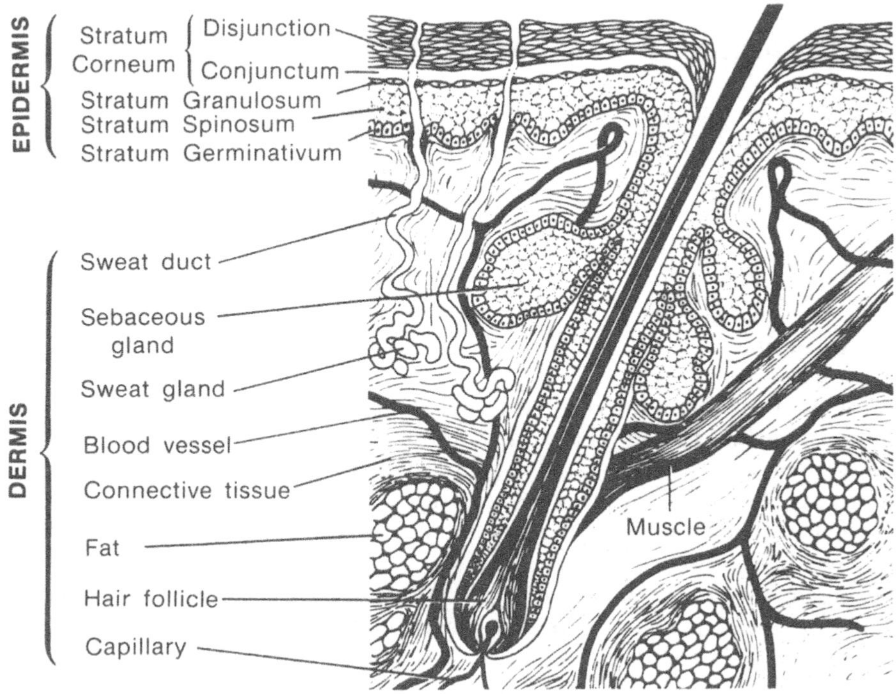

Fig. 1. Schematic diagram of a cross-section of skin. (From [3])

follicles, sebaceous glands, eccrine sweat glands, and apocrine sweat glands. Sweat glands and lipids secreted by the sebaceous glands into the hair follicles help maintain the skin pH at about 5 and can affect adhesion of transdermal systems.

Permeability

In the 1960s, Scheuplein and colleagues began systematic investigations of skin permeability. They used excised specimens of skin in diffusion chambers to study movement of chemicals through skin, and verified that the mechanism is primarily diffusion. The variation in thickness of the stratum corneum was identified as the primary reason for differences in permeation at different anatomic sites [6].

With data from an in vitro test method using cadaver whole skin, epidermis, or dermis mounted as membranes in a diffusion chamber, Michaels, Chandrasekaran, and Shaw [4] created a mathematical model to describe penetration through both lipid and protein phases of the stratum corneum.

Skin Site

While percutaneous absorption of some drugs (e.g., scopolamine) is dependent upon the anatomical site [8, 7], the percutaneous absorption of fentanyl is independent of skin site. In vitro experiments have demonstrated that the cutaneous permeability of fentanyl is essentially the same between the chest, abdomen, and thigh [5]. When TTS (fentanyl) systems were applied to samples of cadaver skin obtained from various sites of the upper body of the same individual, transcutaneous fentanyl flux remained essentially the same among different sites.

Skin Blood Flow

After a drug molecule passes through the skin, it is taken up by local blood vessels that move it to the general circulation. Thus, from a physiological perspective, the appearance of the drug in the systemic circulation is governed not just by the skin permeability but also by the local blood flow.

The skin permeability constant of fentanyl is calculated to be 0.0125 ml/h cm^2 [4]. Because the blood supply to a chest skin site ranges from 0.0122 to 0.0224 ml/min cm^2 [1] the blood flow is 60- to 120-fold that of the fentanyl permeability constant. Therefore, the permeation of fentanyl through the skin appears to be a much slower process than would be permitted by the local blood supply under normal physiological conditions. Only extreme conditions, such as the blood supply to the skin under the system being completely cut off, would influence fentanyl absorption.

Skin Metabolism

For drugs delivered by the transdermal route for systemic therapy, the percutaneous metabolism could be significant because the drug molecule has to pass through the skin before appearing in the systemic circulation. The skin is known to have a broad spectrum of metabolic capacities including phase I reactions (such as oxidation, reduction, and hydrolysis) and phase II reactions (such as glucuronide formation, sulfate formation, and glutathione conjugation). Therefore, the possibility that skin metabolizes fentanyl was examined. Witham and colleagues [11] incubated fentanyl with skin homogenates and found insignificant metabolism of fentanyl. When fentanyl was incubated with skin keratinocytes in vitro, no fentanyl metabolism was detected [AZA Corporation data]. In a bioavailability study, 92 % of the dose delivered by TTS (fentanyl) reached the systemic circulation as unchanged fentanyl [10]. Thus, there is no detectable skin metabolism of fentanyl when delivered transdermally.

Irritation and Sensitization

Because skin irritation and contact sensitization have been reported for some currently marketed transdermal systems, we measured the incidence of topical reactions to TTS (fentanyl). In the studies of cancer patients, 22 (14%) reported sweating, six (4%) reported pruritus, six (4%) reported an application site reaction, two reported rash, and one reported exfoliative dermatitis. There were no reports of sensitization. The incidence of topical irritation in postoperative patients was extremely low: 24 h after TTS (fentanyl) removal, none had edema and fewer than 5% had any local irritation including erythema, papules, pustules, and itching. There were no reports of contact sensitization in postoperative patients.

Effect of Physicochemical Properties of the Drug

Drug Selection

A comparison of the physicochemical properties of fentanyl and morphine illustrates some of the initial information required for selecting a drug candidate for a transdermal system (Table 1).

Because the skin acts like an organic phase, the partitioning of a drug between the skin and the reservoir solution is more in favor of a lipophilic drug. Although the drugs have similiar pKa values, fentanyl is much more lipophilic than morphine, as reflected by the difference in aqueous solubility and as evidenced by fentanyl's larger partition coefficient between octanol and water. Because the diffusion coefficient is dependent upon the molecular weight of the drug, fentanyl and morphine have similar diffusion coefficients.

Despite similar diffusion coefficients in skin, fentanyl has a far more favorable transdermal flux because of large differences in lipophilicity or partition coefficients. The skin flux for fentanyl is 0.26 $\mu g/cm^2$ h, far greater than the 0.006 $\mu g/cm^2$ h value for morphine. Evaluation of more samples has,

Table 1. Physicochemical properties of fentanyl and morphine

	Fentanyl	Morphine
Molecular weight	285.3	336.5
pKa	8.43	8.9
Aqueous solubility of free base	9.9 µg/ml	250 µg/ml
Octanol/water coefficient at pH 7.4	717	0.70
Estimated partition coefficient between skin and water	145	0.29
Diffusion coefficient in skin	$2.4 \times 10^{-11} cm^2/s$	$8.9 \times 10^{-12} cm^2/s$

in fact, revealed that 1 μg/cm² h is a more representative fentanyl skin flux value. Being a much more potent narcotic than morphine, fentanyl is a preferable drug candidate for transdermal delivery because smaller amounts of the drug have to cross the skin to attain similar analgesic effects. However, additional factors need to be considered before fentanyl can be regarded as a safe and effective transdermal product. One important factor is the therapeutically effective dose, or dosing rate. In order to deliver fentanyl at an effective dose, a system size of approximately 10–40 cm² was needed to simply place a saturated fentanyl base solution on the skin.

Rate Control by the System

The approach of using a saturated fentanyl base solution to provide continuous transdermal delivery of fentanyl would rely upon the skin as the sole determinant of drug delivery rate. Because of potential permeability variations among individuals, and among skin sites on the same individual, a special rate-controlling membrane is used in the system to provide additional control of the drug release. If the drug release flux from a therapeutic system into a sink condition is J_{sys}, and the drug flux through the skin when the drug solution is directly placed on the skin is J_{skin}, then the drug flux from the system to the patient when the system is placed on the skin, J_{net}, is defined by the following equation:

$$1/J_{net} = 1/J_{sys} + 1/J_{skin}$$

If the drug release rate from the system is much smaller than J_{skin}, then the net drug flux is essentially the same as J_{sys}, and the system controls the drug flux. On the other hand, if the drug release from the system is much faster than J_{skin}, then the net drug flux is the same as J_{skin}, and the skin controls drug flux. Because J_{skin} varies between individuals, it is only possible to control J_{sys}, and the drug released from the system is much more reproducible under this system-controlled situation. For a delivery system that is system-controlled, the J_{sys} has to be much lower than J_{skin}. The resulting low drug flux may make it impractical to deliver the drug at a therapeutically effective rate with a reasonably sized system. Thus, the final design of TTS (fentanyl) is an optimization between the need to achieve a targeted delivery rate and the need to minimize the subject-to-subject variability in the skin permeability. The rate-controlled delivery of fentanyl reduces the variation in skin drug transport rate by 50%.

As mentioned above, the J_{sys} value needs to be less than the value for J_{skin} in order to impose more system control than skin control on the rate of drug release. Thus the extent of rate control possible is somewhat limited by the need to deliver the drug at a therapeutically effective rate. This limitation can be overcome by using an absorption enhancer to increase the skin drug flux. As the extent of the system control is determined by the ratio of J_{sys} and J_{skin}, the absolute value of J_{skin} is of no consequence to the extent of system control.

We selected alcohol because of its safety record and the ability of a small amount of alcohol to enhance skin permeability of fentanyl. This made it possible to achieve a less variable delivery system while maintaining a reasonably sized system.

TTS (Fentanyl) System Design

ALZA Corporation has developed a Transdermal Therapeutic System [TTS (fentanyl)] providing continuous controlled systemic delivery of fentanyl base for 72 h. It is a rectangular transparent unit comprising a protective peel strip and four functional layers. Proceeding from the outer surface toward the surface adhering to skin, these layers are:

a) a backing layer of polyester film,
b) a drug reservoir of fentanyl and alcohol USP gelled with hydroxyethyl cellulose,
c) an ethylene-vinyl acetate copolymer membrane that controls the rate of fentanyl delivery to the skin surface, and
d) a silicone adhesive. The protective peel strip is removed before use (Fig. 2).

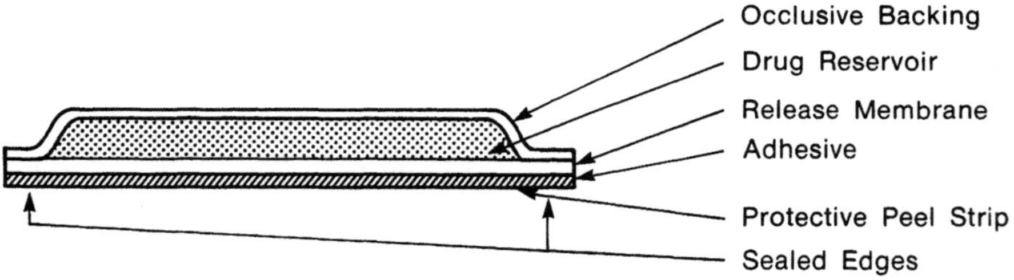

Fig. 2. Cross-section of TTS (fentanyl) system (not to scale)

The amount of fentanyl released from each system (25 μg/h 10 cm^2) is proportional to the surface area (Table 2). Each system also contains a small amount of alcohol (0.1 m/10 cm^2 of system size); a fraction of the alcohol is released during use.

Table 2. Description of TTS (fentanyl) systems

Dose (μg/h)	Size (cm^2)	Fentanyl content (mg)
25	10	2.5
50	20	5
75	30	7.5
100	40	10

When the system is applied the drug initially partitions from the drug-saturated adhesive into the skin. Fentanyl in the adhesive layer permits a priming dose of fentanyl at the start of therapy. This helps to shorten the time required to achieve a given plasma drug concentration because the priming dose hastens the process of establishing the drug concentration gradient in the skin. The priming dose allows the gradient to build up more quickly so that systemic drug input from the system reservoir is more rapid. The skin absorbs fentanyl, and a depot of fentanyl concentrates in the upper skin layers. After diffusion through the skin, fentanyl becomes available to the systemic circulation. Because of this process, fentanyl concentrations are not measurable until 2 h after application.

In addition to understanding the transdermal permeation of a drug, detailed information of its rate-controlled pharmacology is also essential to develop a safe and effective transdermal system.

References

1. Altman PL, Dittmer DS (eds) (1970) Biology data book, 2nd ed. Federation of American Societies for Experimental Biology, Bethesda, Maryland, p 1709 (vol III)
2. Feldmann RJ, Maibach HI (1967) Regional variation in percutaneous penetration of ^{14}C cortisol in man. J Invest Dermatol 48: 181–183
3. Klaassen CD, Amdur MO, Doull J (1986) Casarett and Doull's toxicology: the basic science of poisons, 3rd ed. Macmillan Publishing Company, New York, p 414
4. Michaels AS, Chandrasekaran SK, Shaw JE (1975) Drug permeation through human skin: theory and in vitro experimental measurement. Am Inst Chem Eng 21: 985–996
5. Roy SD, Flynn GL (1990) Transdermal delivery of narcotic analgesics: pH, anatomical, and subject influences on cutaneous permeability of fentanyl and sufentanil. Pharm Res 7(8): 842–847
6. Scheuplein RJ, Blank IH (1971) Permeability of the skin. Physiol Rev 51: 702–747
7. Shaw JE (1982) Transdermal therapeutic systems. In: Brandau R, Lippold BH (eds) Dermal and Transdermal Absorption (1st International Symposium, 12–14 January, 1981, Munich)
8. Shaw JE, Chandrasekaran SK (1981) Transdermal therapeutic systems. In: Prescott LF, Nimmo WS (eds) Drug Absorption. ADIS Press, Balgowlah, Australia, pp 186–193
9. Tauber U (1982) Metabolism of drugs on and in the skin. In: Brandau R, Lippold BH (eds) Dermal and Transdermal Absorption (1st International Symposium, 12–14 January, 1981, Munich)
10. Varvel JR, Shafer SL, Hwang SS, Coen PA, Stanski DR (1989) Absorption characteristics of transdermally administered fentanyl. Anesthesiology 70: 928–934
11. Witham SL, Roy SD, Huang AC, Flynn GL (1986) Concepts in transdermal delivery of narcotics I: Enzymatic activity in the hairless mouse skin and human epidermal homogenates. Pharm Res 3: 54S

Transdermal Therapeutic Systems in Clinical Use: Development and Applications

W. S. NIMMO

Introduction

A drug delivery system may be defined as any drug-containing preparation or dosage form that releases one or more drugs continuously at a predetermined pattern for a fixed period of time. Transdermal systems are delivery systems with the following potential advantages over conventional dosage forms:

1. Prolonged duration of action of a drug with a short half-life
2. Reduced toxicity (local or systemic)
3. Maximum efficacy
4. Selectivity of drug action
5. Reduced frequency of administration
6. Improved compliance
7. Avoidance of first-pass loss that is seen after oral administration of some drugs
8. Absorption independent of environment conditions

Transdermal drug delivery was achieved first using conventional formulations such as ointments and creams. Because skin permeability varies over different parts of the body and because the dosage (concentration of drug × area of application) was not easy to control or reproduce, delivery systems were designed for better control of the rate and duration of drug input.

Systems are available to deliver a drug over a period of 1–7 days. Hyoscine, nitroglycerin, clonidine, estradiol, testosterone, fentanyl, and timolol have been studied clinically.

Hyoscine (0.5 mg over a 3-Day Period)

Hyoscine is an antimuscarinic used to prevent nausea and vomiting associated with motion, radiotherapy and surgery. Conventional dosage forms cause drowsiness, confusion, and blurred vision, and have a relatively short duration of action. Transdermal administration with rate-controlled delivery may prolong the beneficial effect and minimize the adverse effects. Early clinical trials at sea demonstrated prevention of motion-induced nausea in 75 % of susceptible subjects who wore a transdermal system [34, 44].

In patients undergoing minor gynecological surgery, transdermal hyoscine reduced the incidence of postoperative vomiting from 68 % to 42 % in the first 24 h after surgery [42]. In the second and third 24-h periods, there were no differences between the groups. Visual disturbances were more common in the treated group at 48 h (42 % compared with 0 % in the placebo group). In the 72-h period of the study, all patients receiving placebo and 13 of the treated patients (68 %) experienced severe nausea or vomiting. It seems likely that some tolerance to the antiemetic effects of the hyoscine occurred. This has also been reported in laboratory-induced motion sickness [17].

In a comparison of transdermal and intramuscular (im) hyoscine, sedation was greater with im administration while the incidence of nausea and vomiting was similar in both groups [22]. In children, there was no improvement in the incidence of nausea and vomiting but five of the 24 children experienced agitation or hallucinations preoperatively [16].

In addition to these adverse effects, as many as two-thirds of patients experienced dry mouth [4]. In two studies [20, 44] skin irritation occurred in approximately 17 % of patients. This reaction disappeared rapidly on removal of the system.

Glyceryl Trinitrate (Nitroglycerin) (2.5, 5, 10, or 15 mg over 24 h)

Nitrates produce vasodilation when concentrations are high enough in the walls of arteries and veins [21]. They are used in the prophylaxis of angina.

Glyceryl trinitrate is used in a sublingual dosage form from which it is absorbed rapidly, with therapeutic blood concentrations achieved within 2 min. [2].

Transdermal systems produce blood concentrations which are in the same range as those achieved after sublingual dosing. However, tolerance of the effects of nitrates develops rapidly with continuous administration [1, 8, 30, 35, 41]. Both the hemodynamic effects and antianginal activity are reduced, and duration of action of the drug is shortened.

Fluctuating nitrate concentrations and a nitrate-free interval may prevent the development of tolerance of the antianginal action [31].

There may be a "cutaneous first pass" loss of nitroglycerin [18]. In monkeys, 15 %–20 % of nitroglycerin administered transdermally is metabolized during the drug's passage through the skin. It is not yet known if this occurs in humans. However, nitroglycerin may be metabolized significantly by skin surface microflora [9] and this may reduce steady state concentrations.

In a trial of exercise-induced angina, transdermal nitroglycerin applied daily for one week reduced the frequency of attacks [27] but only 56 % of subjects had any response at any time. In a postmarketing surveillance study of 5 mg/day nitroglycerin in 2461 patients with angina, the drug was judged effective in 81 % of patients [5]. Thirty per cent experienced side effects.

Reasons for withdrawal from treatment included headache (5.7 %), other side effects (3.6 %) and failure of therapy (3.1 %).

In a trial in 427 men with a minimum of 3 months' history of chronic stable angina inadequately controlled on beta-blockers alone, continuous use of 5 mg/day nitroglycerin showed no advantage over placebo in terms of efficacy (anginal attacks and sublingual nitroglycerin consumption) or quality of life (measured by a health index of disability) [15]. Headache was more frequent on the active drug and 11 patients withdrew because of this, compared with one in the placebo group.

Thus, transdermal nitroglycerin systems have an antianginal effect for 8–12 h after application, but sustained therapy seems to be ineffective because of tolerance [7, 13].

Clonidine (0.1, 0.2, 0.3 mg/Day for 7 Days)

Clonidine is an alpha-adrenoreceptor agonist used in the treatment of hypertension. It has been available in oral dosage form for 20 years [37]. The transdermal preparation was developed to minimize adverse effects, such as dry mouth and drowsiness, which are thought to be dependent on the high peak plasma concentrations seen after oral dosage, and to provide steady state concentrations for a 7-day period. The oral dosage form has to be taken 2- to 3-times daily.

Transdermal clonidine produces steady-state concentrations on day 3. There may be a depot in the stratum corneum [38]. After removal of the system, plasma concentrations remain constant for 8 h and then decline over 3 days with a mean half-life of 21 h. This half-life is much longer than that seen after oral administration [25]. Approximately 50 % of an administered dose of clonidine is eliminated unchanged by the kidney. In the presence of renal failure, the half-life may be prolonged to more than 40 h [24].

Maximum reduction of arterial pressure is achieved 2 to 3 days after initial application and maintained for at least 7 days or until the system is removed. Then arterial pressure returns to pretreatment values over 3 to 4 days. A sustained reduction in heart rate does not occur during therapy, and the severe rebound hypertension observed after stopping oral clonidine abruptly has not occurred after discontinuing transdermal clonidine [45].

The adverse effects of clonidine are changed by giving the drug transdermally [26]. Dry mouth and somnolence are less frequent during transdermal therapy than with oral therapy, but skin irritation is more common [12]. The reaction in the skin may be severe enough to necessitate stopping the transdermal therapy. Reported incidence of irritation varies from 5 % to 35 % [37].

Estradiol (20, 50, or 100 μg/Day for 3 to 4 Days)

A transdermal preparation of 17 beta-estradiol is used to treat symptoms associated with the menopause. Oral estrogen has been used for 20 years for this purpose but dose-related adverse effects have been a problem. Up to 30 % of an oral dose is metabolized to estrone and other metabolites within the gastrointestinal tract wall or the liver. Partly to compensate for this, high oral doses are given. These result in high peak concentrations of estradiol, and estradiol:estrone ratios of less than 1:1. High concentrations of estrogens in the portal circulation may elevate certain hepatic proteins which, in turn, may cause hypertension, hyperlipidemia, gall bladder disease and thrombosis. Transdermal systems may reduce these effects.

In a crossover study of oral and transdermal estradiol, the transdermal system produced plasma estradiol concentrations similar to those seen in the early follicular phase in premenopausal women. Estrone concentrations rose only slightly and the estradiol:estrone ratio was approximately 1 compared with 0.2 with the oral preparation [33]. After removal of the system, concentrations returned to pretreatment values in 24 h. Continuous application for 3 weeks did not lead to estradiol accumulation whereas, after only three oral doses, there were signs of estrogen retention.

Chetkowski and colleagues [6] compared the physiological effects of transdermal estradiol with oral estrogens in premenopausal and postmenopausal women. Oral estrogens increased the concentrations of circulating renin substrate and several hormone-binding globulins whereas transdermal estradiol did not. The use of either preparation resulted in lower gonadotrophin concentrations, more normal vaginal cells and lowered urinary calcium excretion – all desired effects.

In a comparison of transdermal and oral estrogens over 6 weeks, postmenopausal symptoms and adverse effects did not differ significantly between the groups [32]. Skin irritation occurred in 20 % of patients using the transdermal system.

Transdermal estradiol is as effective as oral estrogens in relieving some of the symptoms of the menopause. It may have fewer undesirable effects than oral administration [23].

Testosterone (5, 10, or 15 mg over 24 h)

Transdermal testosterone preparations have been developed to treat testosterone deficiency in men. In a study by Findlay et al. [14], three sizes of system (containing 5, 10, or 15 mg of the drug) were applied to the skin of the scrotum for 22 h each day for 7 days. Concentrations were in the normal adult male range after application of the 10- or 15-mg systems.

In a study of nine healthy volunteers and seven hypogonadal men [3] there were no biochemical or hematological abnormalities. Patients reported improved well-being and improved sexual function, as indicated by the frequency of erection and ejaculations. There was some transient local itching but no skin irritation.

Fentanyl (25, 50, or 100 μg/h over 1 to 3 Days)

Pain after surgery is commonly treated with intermittent opioids but this regimen is ineffective because of infrequent drug administration and variable drug absorption. Rate-controlled intravenous (i.v.) infusions have improved pain relief [29].

Fentanyl is a potent synthetic opioid in a transdermal system which releases 25, 50, or 100 μg/h for 24- to 72 h [28, 11, 19].

Timolol (30 or 60 mg over 30 h)

Timolol is a beta-adrenoreceptor-blocker which has a short half-life and is subject to extensive first-pass loss. Early clinical studies have shown that it is absorbed across the skin and lowers systolic pressure [43].

Bupranolol (30 mg over 24 h)

This rapidly eliminated beta-adrenoreceptor-blocker may be given transdermally in a system which delivers 30 mg over 24 h. A clinical effect has been demonstrated by a reduction in exercise tachycardia [46].

Azatadine

This antihistamine may be used to reduce histamine-induced wheals and was as effective transdermally as orally in a crossover study in 23 subjects. Both active treatments were better than placebo [10].

Conclusion

Transdermal systems have had some success but not without some problems of tolerance and skin toxicity. Each system must be judged on its own clinical merits and clinical efficacy, and safety cannot be assumed from early blood concentration data alone.

References

1. Abrams J (1986) Tolerance to organic nitrates. Circulation 74: 1181–1185
2. Armstrong PW, Armstrong JA, Marks GS (1979) Blood levels after sublingual nitroglycerin. Circulation 59: 585–588

3. Bals-Pratsch M, Yoon YD, Knuth UA, Nieschlag E (1986) Transdermal testosterone substitution therapy for male hypogonadism. Lancet 2: 943–946
4. Barry BW (1987) Transdermal drug delivery. In: Johnson P, Lloyd-Jones JG (eds) Drug delivery systems. VCH, Chichester, pp 200–223
5. Bridgman KM, Carr M, Tattersal AB (1984) Postmarketing surveillance of the Transderm-Nitro patch in general practice. J Int Med Res 12: 40–45
6. Chetkowski RJ, Meldrum DR, Steingold KA, Randle D, Lu JK, et al. (1986) Biologic effects of transdermal estradiol. N Eng J Med 314: 1615–1620
7. Cowan C, Bourke J, Read DS, Julian DG (1987) Tolerance to glyceryl trinitrate patches: prevention by intermittent dosing. Br Med J 294: 544–545
8. Cowan JC (1986) Nitrate tolerance. Int J Cardiol 12: 1–19
9. Denyer SP, Guy RH, Hadgraft J, Hugo WB (1985) The microbial degradation of topically applied drugs. Int J Pharmaceut 26: 89–97
10. Dietz AJ, Carlson JD, Beck CL (1986) Effect of transdermal azatadine on reducing histamine-induced wheal area. Ann Allergy 57: 38–41
11. Duthie DJR, Rowbotham DJ, Wyld R, Henderson PD, Nimmo WS (1988) Plasma fentanyl concentrations during transdermal delivery of fentanyl to surgical patients. Br J Anaesth 60: 614–618
12. Editorial (1987) Transdermal antihypertensive drugs. Lancet 1: 79–80
13. Editorial (1988) Pharmacological adaptive responses to drugs, Lancet 2: 25–26
14. Findlay JC, Place VA, Snyder PJ (1987) Transdermal delivery of testosterone. J Clin Endocr Metab 64: 266–268
15. Fletcher A, McLoone P, Bulpitt C (1988) Quality of life on angina therapy: a randomised controlled trial of transdermal glyceryl trinitrate against placebo. Lancet 2: 4–8
16. Gibbons PA, Nicolson SC, Betts EK, Rosenberry KR, Jobes DR (1984) Scopolamine does not prevent postoperative emesis after pediatric eye surgery. Anesthesiology 61: A435
17. Greybiel A, Cranmer DB, Wood CD (1982) Anti-motion sickness efficacy of scopolamine 12 and 72 hours after transdermal administration. Aviation Space Environ Med 53: 770–772
18. Guy RH, Hadgraft J, Bucks DAW (1987) Transdermal drug delivery and cutaneous metabolism. Xenobiotica 17: 325–343
19. Holley FO, van Steennis C (1988) Postoperative analgesia with fentanyl: pharmacokinetics and pharmacodynamics of constant rate iv and transdermal delivery. Br J Anaesth 60: 608–613
20. Homick JL, Kohl RL, Reschke MF, Degionanni J, Cintron-Trevino NM (1983) Transdermal scopolamine in the prevention of motion sickness: evaluation of the time course of efficacy. Aviation Space Environ Med 54: 994–1000
21. Imhof PR (1984) Anti-anginal therapy with transdermal nitroglycerin. In: Prescott LF and Nimmo WS (eds) Rate control in drug therapy, Churchill Livingstone, Edinburgh, pp 201–214
22. Jackson SH, Schmitt L, McGuire J, Hall M (1982) Transdermal scopolamine as a preanaesthetic drug, and postoperative antinauseant and antiemetic. Anesthesiology 57: A330
23. Lasagna L, Greenblatt DJ (1986) More than skin deep: transdermal drug-delivery systems. N Eng J Med 314: 1638–1639
24. Lowenthal DT, Matzek KM, MacGregor TR (1988) Clinical pharmacokinetics of clonidine. Clin Pharmacokin 14: 287–310
25. MacGregor TR, Matzek KM, Keirns JJ, van Wayjen RGA, van den Ende A, et al. (1985) Pharmacokinetics of transdermally delivered clonidine. Clinical Pharmacol Ther 38: 278–284
26. McMahon FG, Michael R, Jain A, Ryan JR (1984) Clinical experience with clonidine TTS. In: Weber and Mathias (eds) Mild Hypertension, Steinkopff, Darmstadt pp 148–152

27. Muiesan G, Agabiti-Rosei E, Muiesen L, Romanelli G, Pollavini P et al (1986) A multicenter trial of transdermal nitroglycerin in exercise-induced angina: individual antianginal response after repeated administration. Am Heart J 112: 223–238
28. Nimmo WS, Duthie DJR (1986) Plasma fentanyl concentrations after transdermal or iv infusion of fentanyl. Anesthesiology 65: A559
29. Nimmo WS, Todd JG (1985) Fentanyl by constant rate iv infusion for postoperative analgesia. Br J Anaest 57: 250–254
30. Packer M, Medina N, Yushak M, Lee WH (1986) Hemodynamic factors limiting the response to transdermal nitroglycerin in severe chronic congestive heart failure. Am J Cardiol 57: 260–267
31. Parker JO, Fung H-L (1984) Transdermal nitroglycerin in angina pectoris. Am J Cardiol 54: 471–476
32. Place VA, Powers MS, Darley PE, Schenkel L, Good WR (1985) A double blind comparative study of Estraderm and Premarin in the amelioration of postmenopausal symptoms. Am J Obstet Gyn 152: 1092–1099
33. Powers MS, Schenkel L, Darley PE, Good WR, Balestra JC, et al. (1985) Pharmacokinetics and pharmacodynamics of transdermal dosage forms of 17 beta-estradiol: comparison with conventional oral estrogens used for hormone replacement. Am J Obstet Gyn 152: 1099–1106
34. Price NM, Schmitt LG, McGuire J, Shaw JE, Trobough G (1981) Transdermal scopolamine in the prevention of motion sickness at sea. Clin Pharmacol Ther 29: 414–419
35. Reichek N, Goldstein RE, Redwood DR, Epstein SE (1974) Sustained effects of nitroglycerin ointment in patients with angina pectoris. Circulation 50: 348–352
36. Reiniger G, Menke G, Boertz A, Kraus F, Rudolph W (1987). Interval treatment for an effective therapy of angina pectoris with transdermal nitroglycerin patches. Herz 12: 68–73
37. Ridout G, Santus G, Guy RH (1988) Pharmacokinetic considerations in the use of newer transdermal formulations. Clin Pharmacokin 15: 114–131
38. Shaw JE (1984) Pharmacokinetics of nitroglycerin and clonidine delivered by the transdermal route. Am Heart J 108: 217–223
39. Shaw JE, Chandrasekaran SK (1981) Transdermal therapeutic systems. In: Prescott LF, Nimmo WS (eds) Drug Absorption. ADIS Press, New York 186–193
40. Shaw JE, Theeuwes F (1984) Transdermal dosage forms. In: Prescott LF, Nimmo WS (eds) Rate control in drug therapy. Churchill Livingstone, Edinburgh, pp 65–70
41. Thadani U, Hamilton SF, Olson E, Anderson J, Voyles W, et al. (1986) Transdermal nitroglycerin patches in angina pectoris. Ann Intern Med 105: 485–492
42. Uppington J, Dunnet J, Blogg CE (1986) Transdermal hyoscine and postoperative nausea and vomiting. Anaesthesia 41: 16–20
43. Vlasses PH, Ribeiro LGT, Rotmensch HH, Bondi JV, Loper AE, et al. (1985) Initial evaluation of transdermal timolol: serum concentrations and beta-blockade. J Cardiovasc Pharmacol 7: 245–250
44. von Marion WF, Bogaert MG, Christiaanse JC, Hofkamp HG, van Ouwerkark W (1985) Influence of transdermal scopolamine on motion sickness during 7 days exposure to heavy seas. Clin Pharmacol Ther 38: 301–305
45. Weber MA, Drayer J (1984) Clinical experience with rate controlled delivery of antihypertensive therapy by a transdermal system. Am Heart J 108: 231–236
46. Wellstein A, Kuppers H, Pitscher HF, Palm D (1986) Transdermal delivery of bupranolol: pharmacodynamics and beta-adrenoreceptor occupancy. Eur J Clin Pharmacol 31: 419–422

Part II. Current Aspects of Pain Management

Postoperative Pain

K. A. LEHMANN, S. GROND, and D. ZECH

Arguments for Postoperative Pain Management

Nowadays many patients are not so worried about anesthesia as about the first few hours following surgery. Although the need for reliable postoperative monitoring of the cardiovascular or respiratory systems is universally accepted, the call for similar attention in the field of analgesia is mostly met by ignorance. The most important task of anesthesiologists is the relief of pain. We anesthesiologists not only provide surgeons with comfortable and safe operating conditons, but should equally feel bound, for ethical reasons, to help patients with their postanesthetic complaints. This argument ("compassion") seems to be too often neglected in clinical practice.

Notwithstanding, there are important medical reasons for alleviation of pain. Pain induces autonomic reactions which are undesirable in the early postoperative period. Signs of increased sympathetic tone include hypertension, tachycardia, or sweating; these symptoms, however, are not pain-specific since they may also be found in hypothermia, hypovolemia, hypercapnia, or hypoxia. The same is true for stress-induced endocrine reactions which consequently cannot be used as reliable indicators of pain.

Pain often impedes effective physiotherapy or respiratory exercises which in turn may lead to an increase in postoperative complications (pneumonias, thromboses, emboli, etc.) [18, 42]. However, whether reconvalescence can really be influenced by the quality of pain treatment is controversial; the literature contains positive [4, 20, 89, 126, 131] as well as negative reports [35, 48, 100, 120].

The outcome of postoperative pain treatment is often described as insufficient. Unfortunately, there are only a few thorough surveys available [14, 16, 27, 60, 64, 82, 87, 98, 134] which mostly blame poor knowledge among physicians and the nursing staff with respect to basic pain physiology or pharmacology. On the other hand, it is our personal opinion that a reasonable *feedback* between patients and therapists is the most urgent requirement for the control of therapeutic outcome, which is undisputably accepted in any other branch of medicine. Figure 1 shows some results of a German survey on postoperative pain management [64]. It is evident from this inquiry that most anesthetists are better informed on laboratory results

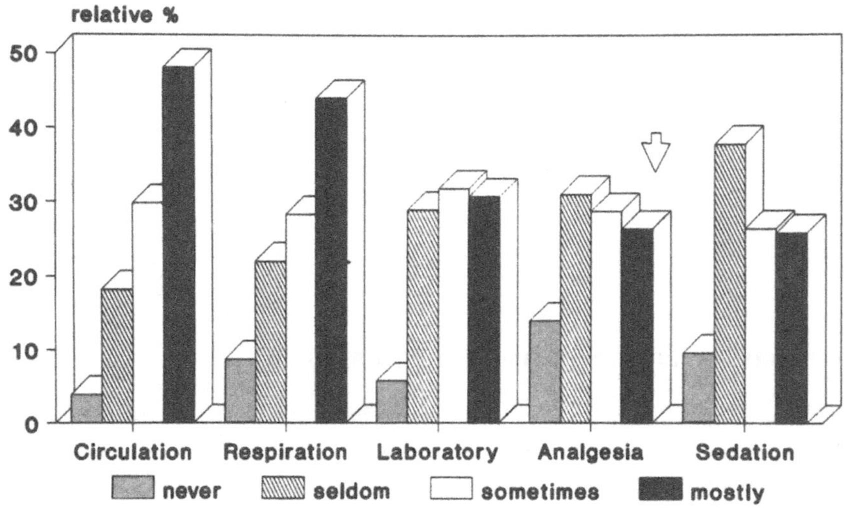

Fig. 1. Anesthetists' information on patients' postoperative status. (From [64])

than about pain! Clearly more time must be spent with postoperative patients in order to improve postoperative analgesia; uncontrolled prescriptions at the end of surgery are inadequate.

Psychological and Physiological Aspects

There are relatively few investigations on *predictors* of postoperative pain, and, since pain is difficult to measure, their results often look contradictory [36, 39, 47, 56, 116]. Although most studies assume that personality factors (anxiety, neuroticism, extroversion, etc.) play a significant role, reliable conclusions are not yet possible for individual patients. Age or gender seems less important, as do premedication or anesthetic techniques, although there are some newer contradictory opinions [12, 21, 85, 87]. This is particularly true if one considers the strong influence of preoperative information on postoperative pain tolerance [28, 30, 116].

It is often stressed that "simple" wound pain is only one aspect of postoperative complaints, and that comfort is also disturbed by anxiety, headache, nausea/vomiting or colic pain [56]. Again, it must be self-evident that adequate (differential) treatment can only be expected if patients are carefully looked after by a physician.

Patient-controlled analgesia (PCA) has undisputably shown that intersubject differences in analgesic needs after surgery are of utmost importance. Figure 2 displays cumulative dose-time plots of 40 postoperative patients who were allowed to self-administer intravenous morphine. While some need virtually no opiate analgesic at all, even after major abdominal surgery, others

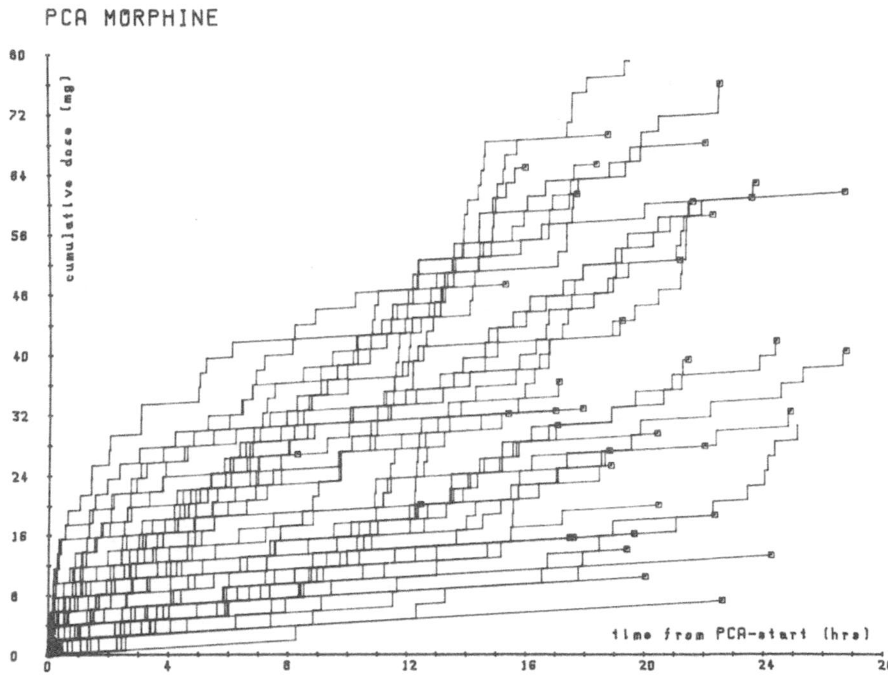

Fig. 2. Postoperative morphine consumption (patient-controlled analgesia, PCA) following major abdominal and orthopedic surgery. (From Lehmann et al., unpublished results)

demand rather high doses after so-called "small" operations like meniscectomies [63]. Since the consumption rates seem to be stable for most patients, it follows from such results that a relatively short observation period in the recovery room (3–4 h) may be the best "predictor" for the first postoperative day – provided the patients really receive the amount of analgesic they actually need during this period.

PCA also proved that age is indeed a predictor of postoperative analgesic needs. As shown in Fig. 3, the cumulative morphine dosage of 120 patients recovering from general surgery was significantly correlated with age. But what do statistics mean to the patient? Indeed, individual differences are large enough to require individual treatment for each patient.

Finally, it became evident from PCA studies that pharmacokinetically calculated predictors of pain are far less important than we anticipated. Figure 4 and Table 1 show minimum effective concentrations (MEC) from several investigations performed by the authors' group [65, 66, 71, 72, 73] and from the literature. Blood samples were taken immediately prior to patients' demand, and opiate plasma concentrations were determined. There was no generalizable "threshold" concentration at which all patients felt pain relief diminish, although we could describe the lower part of the therapeutic

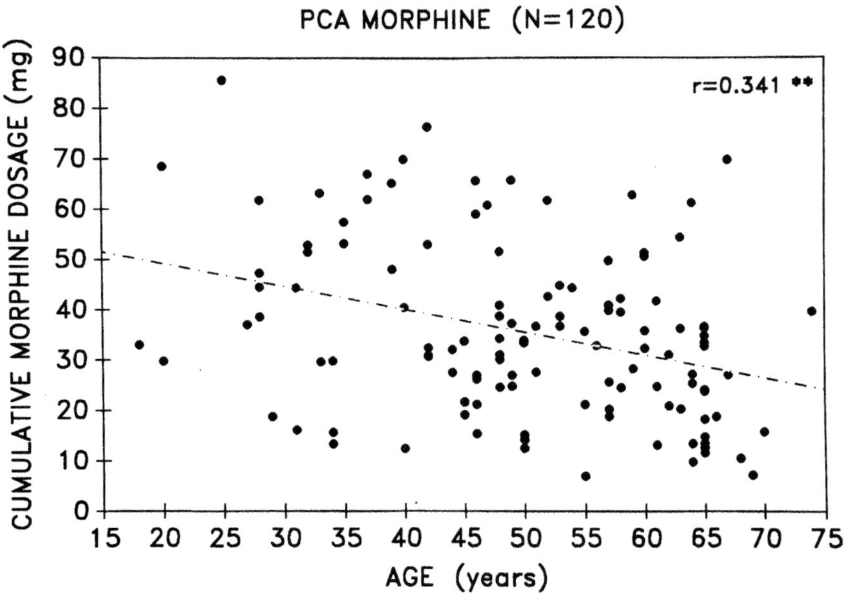

Fig. 3. Correlation of postoperative morphine consumption (PCA) and age following elective surgery. (From Lehmann et al., unpublished results)

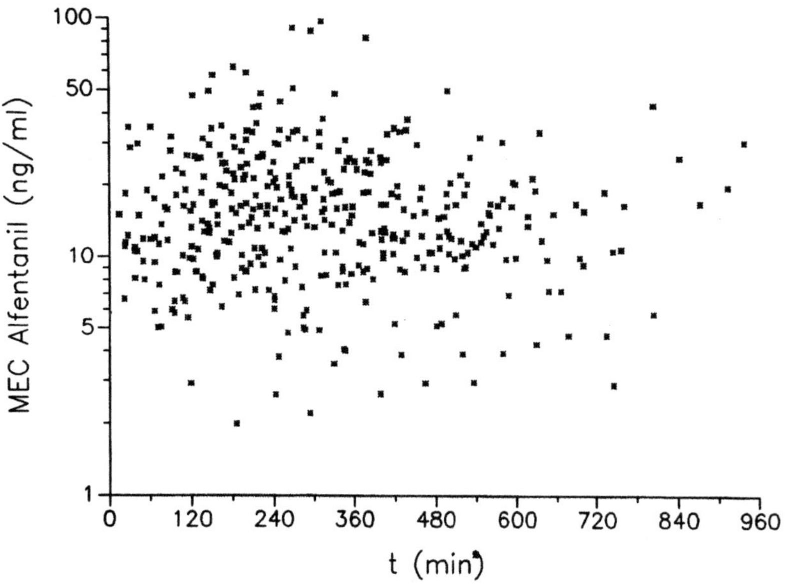

Fig. 4. Postoperative alfentanil, minimum effective concentrations (MEC), based on the duration of PCA treatment [73]

Table 1. Minimum effective concentrations (MEC) during postoperative PCA (results from several studies performed by the authors and from the literature)

Analgesic	Mean MEC	Relative potency based on MEC (Morphine = 1)
Sufentanil	0.04	400
Buprenorphine	0.38	42
Fentanyl	0.63	25
	1.16	14
	1.54	10
Hydrocodone	6	3
Alfentanil	15	1
Morphine	16	1
Ketobemidone	28	0.6
Tramadol	289	0.05
	915	0.02
Pethidine	455	0.04

windows and the medians of concentrations which should be exceeded to provide adequate analgesia.

It would be too easy to assume that the frequency of nociceptive impulses is a reasonable measure of "pain". Clinical pain can be best described as a complex psychophysiological experience which is difficult to quantify. Nevertheless, methods of *algesiometry* are available not only for laboratory evaluations but also for clinical practice [70]. Their precision is limited, of course, but they are an essential prerequisite for the judgement of therapeutic success and thus for the feedback we called for so urgently earlier. As was shown by Jensen et al. [51], verbal or numeric rating scales, as well as visual analogue scales, are equally suitable and easy to handle, whereas multidimensional techniques such as the McGill pain questionnaire are often found too difficult in the early postoperative period. With these tools it is possible to document pain intensities on the patient's record as routinely as blood pressure or pulse rates, which should really be required for all surgical wards. Only if we realize how insufficient pain relief often is, are we likely to reconsider our current strategies.

Methods for Postoperative Pain Treatment

It is now well known that there are at least three targets for analgesic therapy. Antipyretic or antiphlogistic analgesics prevent the stimulation of peripheral nociceptors, local anesthetics inhibit conduction of nociceptive impulses, and centrally acting analgesics (opiates) impede synaptic transmission both on cord and cerebral levels [68].

Systemic Pharmacotherapy

As was shown in one of our own studies, systemic pharmacotherapy represents the most frequently used method of postoperative pain relief, at least in Germany [64]. Among the various drugs available, opiate analgesics are most favored (Fig. 5).

Opiate Analgesics

The modifying effects of opiate analgesics on mood and emotional aspects of pain have been regarded as essential for a long time. Since the discovery of specific opiate receptors and endorphins it has become evident that opiates influence pain transmission as well as autonomic and endocrine reflexes; hence their effects apply to patients suffering from or reacting to pain [41, 69].

Recent research has documented the existence of different types of opiate receptors which may be responsible for the expression of opiate effects (or side effects). Accordingly, opiate analgesics are classified with regard to their extrinsic and intrinsic activities at these specific receptor sites. Most clinically used opiates are μ-receptor agonists. The so-called agonist–antagonists often exert agonistic effects at one receptor type (e.g., κ) while they are antagonists to others (e.g. buprenorphine or nalbuphine). Since the overall number of opiate receptors is limited, the dose-effect curve looks characteristic. If all available receptors are occupied, increasing the dosage no longer leads to an increase of specific effects ("ceiling effect"). Ceiling effects at rather low dosages are particularly known for agonist–antagonists (e.g. pentazocine, nalbuphine or buprenorphine). While this is often claimed (by pharmaceu-

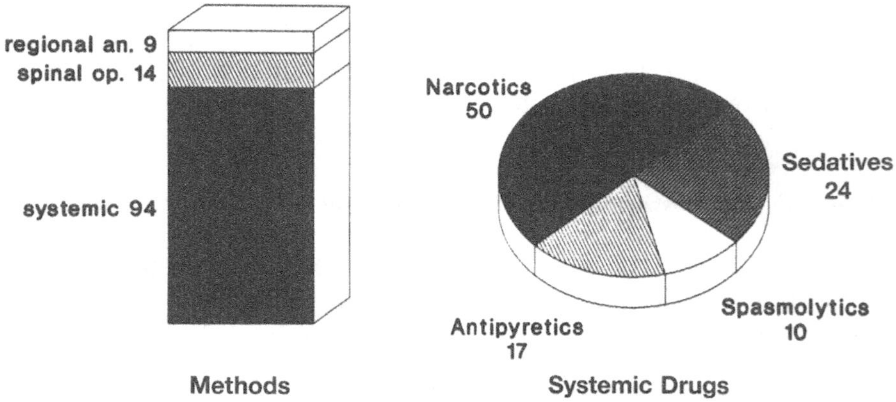

Fig. 5. Methods of postoperative pain management and systemic drugs preferred in Germany [64]

tical companies) to be advantageous with respect to respiratory depression, one should be aware of similar limitations regarding analgesia.

While the danger of tolerance or even dependence hardly ever restricts the use of postoperative opiates, *respiratory depression* may be a problem. It is mainly mediated by a reduced sensitivitiy of central chemoreceptors and manifests itself as a decreased or even absent respiratory drive, which can usually be overcome by commands to breathe. Evidence is accumulating now that clinically relevant respiratory depression is connected to *overdosage* which in turn reduces the problem to adequate dose-finding strategies. If one admits that 10 – 30 % of surgical patients need no postoperative analgesics at all, then even 5 mg morphine intramuscularly may mean overdosage. On the other hand, it could be shown with patient-controlled analgesia that patients demanding "incredibly" high opiate dosages (Table 3) because of very severe pain were never in danger of respiratory depression. Figure 6 shows results of a recent investigation in which postoperative patients were closely monitored for transcutaneous O_2, CO_2 and oxygen saturation. Data were collected every 30 s over a 4 h observation period. There was no evidence that conventionally treated patients were less at respiratory risk than the PCA patients.

Thus the general rule to prevent central respiratory depression must be to administer only that dosage which is individually necessary: this means

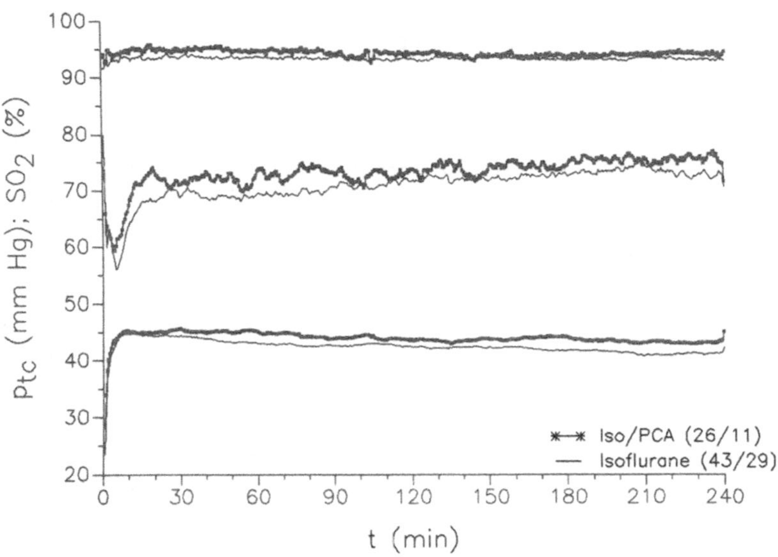

Fig. 6. Results of continuous postoperative respiratory monitoring in two groups of patients recovering from major gynecological surgery performed under isoflurane anesthesia. One group was given conventional intramuscular analgesia on request, the other was allowed to self-administer intravenous opiates.
(Means: *top,* oxygen saturation; *middle,* transcutaneous oxygen; *bottom,* transcutaneous carbon dioxide. Since pulse oximetry was not available at the start of the study, fewer patients were simultaneously monitored for all three variables). (From Lehmann et al., unpublished results)

individual *titration* which can be best performed by i. v. injection. Adequate surveillance must be guaranteed, of course, and naloxone should always be available. It should also be mentioned that buprenorphine is hardly antagonizable by naloxone due to its extremely high receptor binding, and that respiratory analeptics such as doxapram can be necessary in the case of overdosage.

For practical therapy, these considerations are important:
a) choice of analgesic drug, and
b) site and mode of application.

Concerning the *choice of the analgesic drug,* conclusive recommendations are difficult to make. In our own experience all available opiate agonists and most agonist-antagonists are comparably suitable, provided that equipotent, and adequate (!), dosages are used; for this reason we recommend choosing those drugs to which the physicians and the nursing staff are the most accustomed. For the treatment of short-term pain peaks (e.g., changing of wound dressings, mobilization etc.), we prefer drugs with a fast onset and limited duration of action (e.g., alfentanil and fentanyl), whereas we share the opinion of the German inquiry [64] which indicated an order of importance as follows: piritramide (28 %), buprenorphine (24 %), pentazocine (20 %), pethidine (13 %) and tramadol (10 %) for routine pain treatment. It should be mentioned in passing that some authors warn against switching from agonists to agonist–antagonists or vice-versa, and although there may be theoretical reasons to explain such warnings, we are not aware of any convincing clinical data that justify them.

The *site and mode of application* seem more critical. The intramuscular route is obviously preferred, although there are many objections to be made. Absorption is generally very variable, and this is particularly true for postoperative patients with local hypoperfusion as a consequence of hypovolemia or hypothermia. In addition, it usually takes too long until effects become evident, which makes the patients suffer unnecessarily and prevents the therapist from making an early judgement about the therapeutic otucome. Only intravenous bolus injection (or adaptive intravenous infusion) permits titration of the dosage to individual needs. As soon as these needs have been met after an initial physician-controlled period, there is no argument against maintenance therapy by continuous infusion [6, 37, 53, 94, 125] or even by repetitive intramuscular injections at fixed time intervals which can be provided and controlled by the nursing staff. In any event frequent pain measurements and, as a consequence, dose adjustments, must be guaranteed. The same will be true, of course, for transdermally applied opiates.

Recommendations such as those given in Table 2 are necessary, but one must not forget that individual needs are subject to tremendous variability.

PCA obviously fulfills most of the above-mentioned criteria (for reviews see [4, 31, 44, 67]). Success rates are mostly described as convincing to

Table 2. Narcotic analgesics for acute pain treatment (recommendations from the literature)

Drug	Relative potency	Single intravenous dose (mg)	Mean duration of of action (h)
Fentanyl	100–300	0.05–0.1	0.3–0.5
Buprenorphine	40–50	0.15–0.3	6–8
Alfentanil	10–50	0.5–1	0.1–0.2
L-Methadone	2–3	7.5–10	4–8
Morphine	1	5–10	2–5
Piritramide	0.7	7.5–15	3–6
Pentazocine	0.3	30–50	2–5
Pethidine	0.1	50–100	1–4
Tramadol	0.1	50–100	1–4

overwhelming. In our own studies about 75% of the patients who had experienced earlier conventional treatment preferred intravenous self-administration. Most investigators in the field of PCA underline that we can learn from PCA results (and thus from the patients themselves) what is wrong with conventional techniques and how we can improve daily practice – even without expensive infusion pumps. Table 3 displays mean analgesic consumption for several opiates; most dosages appear to be higher than those usually prescribed in conventional postoperative pain treatment.

Table 3. Mean opiate consumption during the first 24 h after general surgery with intravenous PCA (mg/24 h/70 kg) [67]

Sufentanil	0.17	Piritramide	54.6
Fentanyl	0.77	Nalbuphine	197.4
Buprenorphine	1.1	Pentazocine	227.8
Alfentanil	8.3	Pethidine	294.2
L-Methadone	16.8	Tramadol	341.2
Morphine	49.7		

Antipyretic Analgesics

The sensitivity of nociceptors is increased by algogenic mediators among which the prostaglandins are of particular importance. Inhibitors of prostaglandin (or cyclooxygenase) synthesis can therefore be used for pain relief. Most drugs of this series also reduce inflammation and swelling; because of their antipyretic effects they are classified as antipyretic (antiphlogistic) analgesics. Although some textbooks address them as peripherally acting analgesics, there is increasing evidence that some effects are also mediated at central sites of action, and it is certainly misleading to call them mild analgesics because certain types of pain (like headache or arthritic pain) react to antipyretic analgesics better than to opiates. Unfortunately, postoperative pain is seldom of such an etiology or intensity that antipyretics provide sufficient pain relief [127]. Nevertheless, most compounds have been found useful after minor operations or on the second day after major surgery when wound pain is continuously decreasing.

Common side effects of all NSAIDs (nonsteroidal antiinflammatory drugs) are explained from their inhibition of prostaglandin synthesis. Gastrointestinal irritation is frequently seen, although ulcers hardly develop within the short period of postoperative pain treatment. Allergic reactions may occur (asthmatic episodes following aspirin can be observed in about 1% of previously healthy patients and in about 4% of asthmatics). Some authors believe that impairment of coagulation which regularly takes place with NSAIDs means a general contraindication of these drugs in surgical patients, in particular if simultaneous heparinization is prescribed [17, 106, 114]; there are several clinical studies, however, which do not agree with such conclusions [13, 46, 76, 113].

Table 4 lists some references on the most frequently used antipyretics, while Table 5 gives dose recommendations.

Table 4. Some literature on the postoperative use of antipyretic analgesics

Drug	Reference
ASA[a]	7, 33, 34, 53, 58
Diclofenac	8, 13, 24, 95, 133
Diflunisal	32, 41
Ibuprofen	26, 46, 97
Indomethacin	17, 83, 106, 113
Metamizole[b]	40, 67, 99
Naproxen	81
Paracetamol[c]	11, 46, 76, 102, 109, 114, 124, 135
Piroxicam	7, 86

[a] Acetylsalicylic acid
[b] Dipyrone
[c] Acetaminophen

Drug Combinations

Analgesic drug combinations play an important role in the (self-)treatment of everyday pain, although there are many objections from a pharmacological point of view. The aim is to reduce the dosages of both components in order to reduce the incidence of side effects, but this goal is not always reached [11, 102, 124]. Nevertheless, reduction in opiate consumption has been reported for several *antipyretic analgesics,* e.g., ASA [53], diclofenac [24], ibuprofen

Table 5. Equipotencies and dose recommendations for antipyretic analgesics in the treatment of slight to moderate postoperative pain

Drug	Equipotent dose compared with 650 mg ASA (mg)	Usual single dosage (mg)	Time between doses (h)
ASA[a]	650	600–1000	4
Diflunisal	500	500	12
Indomethacin	25	25–50	8
Fenbufen	400	300–600	12
Fenoprofen	300	300–600	8
Flurbiprofen	100	50–100	8
Ibuprofen	200	200–400	4–6
Naproxen	300	300–600	8
Paracetamol[c]	650	500–1000	4–6
Metamizol[b]		500–1000	4–6

[a] Acetylsalicylic acid
[b] Dipyrone
[c] Acetaminophen

[26, 97], indomethacin [106] or naproxen [81]. Patients recovering from surgery of hollow organs often profit from *spasmolytic agents* (e.g., butylscopolamine, if necessary in combination with metamizole [dipyrone]).

Combinations of opiates with psychotropic drugs are controversial, at least in the treatment of postoperative pain. Neuroleptics of the phenothiazine [29] or butyrophenone [54] type have all been tried, but most studies indicate that they are only of limited value; some authors stress that their antiemetic effects are desirable. Tricyclic antidepressants must be discussed similarly [75]. Benzodiazepines, which are rather often used in the recovery room, may or may not potentiate opiate analgesia [2, 88, 123] but may, by reducing vigilance, enhance respiratory depression. It is certainly a good recommendation to prescribe tranquilizers, if necessary, only after adequate pain treatment with true analgesics.

To summarize, opiates are the drugs of first choice in the systemic treatment of moderate to severe postoperative pain. If they are adequately used (i.e., with individual titration, feedback, and dose adjustment) they prove efficacious and safe. Antipyretics may be added if inflammation or fever become prominent; spasmolytics are helpful in accompanying colic pain states.

Local and regional anesthesia

There is no argument against the usefulness of regional anesthesia for the treatment of postoperative pain [68]. Whenever catheters have been placed

Table 6. Some recent literature on regional anesthetic techniques for the relief of postoperative pain

Technique	References
Wound infiltration	38, 45, 74, 89, 96, 100, 101, 128, 130
Axillary plexus block	1, 80, 104, 111, 129
3-in-1 block	23, 52, 84, 93
Intercostal block	3, 59, 90, 91, 115
Intrapleural infiltration	9, 10, 35, 55, 61, 107, 108, 110, 122, 132
Epidural anesthesia	25, 103, 117, 118, 119

Table 7. Some recent literature on the combination of opiate analgesics and local anesthetics for the relief of postoperative pain

Opiate analgesic	References
Buprenorphine	15, 79, 121
Fentanyl	50, 57, 92, 112
Morphine	5, 19, 21, 22, 43, 49, 62, 77, 78, 136, 137

for intraoperative conduction blocks they should be used as long as possible postoperatively. Since these techniques are of less importance to the present workshop, this review will be restricted to some quotations of interesting newer studies.

Conclusions

This presentation has revealed that effective methods for the control of postoperative pain are available. If they were adequately used, no patient would have to suffer from strong or even exhausting pain. It is our personal impression, however, that this request is all too seldom met.

Strong analgesics are often withheld from postoperative patients because physicians and the nursing staff are afraid of respiratory depression. There is increasing evidence now that opiate-induced respiratory depression will occur only at overdosage. Precisely when an individual postoperative patient will be overdosed cannot easily be predicted. Thus, individual titration must be performed, which is most simply achieved by intravenous injection of small bolus doses. As soon as the individual consumption rate has been determined, prophylactic dosing strategies may be used, but their efficay (and side effects) must be regularly monitored. Postoperative pain is known to decrease significantly during the first 24–48 h after surgery. Thus, any analgesic technique which is not adapted to decreasing needs (or not really adaptable, as we suppose transdermal fentanyl will be) may be potentially dangerous.

Medical therapy always implies diagnosis, treatment and control of therapeutic results. Postoperative pain certainly is a problem requiring therapy. For these reasons, anesthesiologists should feel obliged to act like (all other) physicians – not only during anesthesia but also in the postoperative period. If patients are neglected because of organizational problems, the consequence must be a change of organization – even if that means that more staff are needed for an Acute Pain Service [105] or fewer anesthesias are performed.

References

1. Ang ET, Lassale B, Goldfarb G (1984) Continuous axillary brachial plexus block – a clinical and anatomical study. Anesth Analg 63: 680
2. Artru AA (1986) Midazolam potentiates the analgesic effects of morphine in patients with postoperative pain. Clin J Pain 2: 93
3. Baxter AD, Jennings FO, Harris RS, Flynn JF, Way J (1987) Continuous intercostal blockade after cardiac surgery. Br J Anaesth 59: 162
4. Bennett RL, Griffen WD (1983). Patient-controlled analgesia (PCA): optimization of in-hospital narcotic analgesia therapy. Contemp Surg 23: 75
5. Bisgaard C, Mouridsen P, Dahl JB (1990) Continuous lumbar epidural bupivacaine plus morphine versus epidural morphine after major abdominal surgery. Eur J Anaesth 7: 219
6. Bray RJ (1983) Postoperative analgesia provided by morphine infusion in children. Anaesthesia 38: 1075
7. Breivik H, Stenseth R, Apalseth K, Spilsberg AM (1984) Piroxicam, acetylsalicylic acid and placebo for postoperative pain. Acta Anaethesiol Scand 28: 37
8. Bricker SRW, Savage ME, Hanning CD (1987) Peri-operative blood loss and non-steroidal anti-inflammatory drugs: an investigation using diclofenac in patients undergoing transurethral resection of the prostate. Eur J Anaeth 4: 429
9. Brismar B, Pettersson N, Tokics L, Strandberg A, Hedenstierna G (1987) Postoperative analgesia with intrapleural administration of bupivacaine adrenaline. Acta Anaesthesiol Scand 31: 515
10. Bruce DL, Gerken V, Lyon GD (1987) Postcholecystectomy pain relief by intrapleural bupivacaine in patients with cystic fibrosis. Anesth Analg 66: 1187
11. Bullingham RES, McQuay HJ, Moore RA, Weir L (1981) An oral buprenorphine and paracetamol combination compared with paracetamol alone: A single dose double-blind postoperative study. Br J Clin Pharmacol 12: 863
12. Burns JW, Hodsman NBA, McLintock TTC, Gillies GWA, Kenny GNC, McArdle CS (1989) The influence of patient characteristics on the requirements for postoperative analgesia, A reassessment using patient-controlled analgesia. Anaesthesia 44: 2
13. Carlborg L, Lindoff C, Hellmann A (1987) Diclofenac versus pethidine in the treatment of pain after hysterectomy. Eur J Anaesth 4: 241
14. Cartwright PD (1985) Pain control after surgery: a survey of current practice. Ann R Coll Surg Engl 67: 13
15. Celleno D, Capogna G (1989) Spinal buprenorphine for postoperative analgesia after caesarean section. Acta Anaesthesiol Scand 33: 236
16. Cohen FL (1980) Postsurgical pain relief: patient's status and nurses' medication choices. Pain 9: 265
17. Collier DSJ, Pain JA (1983) Rectal indomethacin for control of postoperative pain. Br Med J 287: 1799
18. Cousins MJ (1989) Acute pain and the injury response: immediate and prolonged effects. Regional Anesthesia 14: 162

19. Cullen ML, Staren ED, El-Ganzouri A, Logas WG, Ivankovich AD, Economou SG (1985) Continuous epidural infusion for analgesia after major abdominal operations: a randomized, prospective, double-blind study. Surgery 98: 718
20. Cuschieri RJ, Morran CG, Howie JC, McArdle CS (1985) Postoperative pain and pulmonary complications: comparison of three analgesic regimes. Br J Surg 72: 495
21. Dahl JB, Rosenberg J, Dirkes WE, Mogensen T, Kehlet H (1990) Prevention of postoperative pain by balanced analgesia. Br J Anaesth 64: 518
22. Dalens B, Tanguy A, Haberer JP (1986) Lumbar epidural anesthesia for operative and postoperative pain relief in infants and young children. Anesth Analg 65: 1069
23. Dalens B, Vanneuville G, Tanguy A (1989) Comparison of the fascia iliaca compartment block with the 3-in-1 block in children. Anesth Analg 69: 705
24. Derbyshire DR, Richardson J (1987) Voltrarol (Diclofenac) as a perioperative analgesic supplement. Br J Anaesth 59: 1373P
25. Desparmet J, Meistelman C, Barre J, Saint-Maurice C (1987) Continuous epidural infusion of bupivacaine for postoperative pain relief in children. Anesthesiology 67: 108
26. Dionne RA, Campbell RA, Cooper SA, Hall DL, Buckingham B (1983) Suppression of postoperative pain by preoperative administration of ibuprofen in comparison to placebo, acetaminophen, and acetaminophen plus codeine. J Clin Pharmacol 23: 37
27. van der Does AJW (1989) Patient's and nurses' ratings of pain and anxiety after burn wound care. Pain 39: 95
28. Donovan BD (1983) Patient attitudes to postoperative pain relief. Anaesth Intensive Care 11: 125
29. Dundee JW, Love WL, Moore J (1963) Alterations in response to somatic pain associated with anaesthesia. XV. Further studies with phenothiazine derivatives and similar drugs. Br J Anaesth 35: 597
30. Egbert LD, Battit GE, Welch CE, Bartlett MK (1964) Reduction of postoperative pain by encouragement and instruction of patients. A study of doctor-patient rapport. N Engl J Med 270: 825
31. Ferrante FM, Ostheimer GW, Covino BG (eds) Patient-controlled analgesia. Blackwell Scientific Publications, Boston 1990
32. Forbes JA, Beaver WT, White EH, White RW, Neilson GB, Shackleford RW (1982) A new oral analgesic with an unusually long duration of action. JAMA 248: 2139
33. Forbes JA, Calderazzo JP, Bowser MW, Foor VM, Shackleford RW, Beaver WT (1982) A 12 hour evaluation of the analgesic efficacy of diflunisal, aspirin and placebo in postoperative dental pain. J Clin Pharmacol 22: 89
34. Foster JMG, Cashman JN, Jones RM (1985) Parenteral aspirin for pain relief in day-case dental anaesthsia. A randomized double blind placebo controlled study. Anaethesia 40: 576
35. Frank ED, McKay W, Rocco A, Gallo JP (1990) Interpleural bupivacaine for postoperative analgesia following cholecystectomy: a randomized prospective study. Regional Anesthesia 15: 26
36. Fraser RA, Hotz SB, Hurtig JB, Hodes SN, Moher D (1989) The prevalence and impact of pain after day-care tubal ligation surgery. Pain 39: 189
37. Fry ENS (1984) Postoperative analgesia: a technique using continuous intravenous infusion of buprenorphine. Anaethesia 39: 1134
38. Gibbs P, Cuschieri RJ (1988) Intermittent wound perfusion. Br J Anaesth 60: 119
39. Gil KM, Ginsberg B, Muir M, Sykes D, Williams DA (1990) Patient-controlled analgesia in postoperative pain: the relation of psychological factors to pain and analgesic use. Clin J Pain 6: 137
40. Gómez-Jiménez J, Fraco-Patino R, Chargoy-Vera J, Olivares-Sosa R (1980) Clinical efficacy of mild analgesics in pain following gynaecological or dental surgery. Br J Clin Pharmacol 10: 355S
41. Gourlay GK, Cousins MJ (1984) Strong analgesics in severe pain. Drugs 28: 79

42. Grond S, Lehmann KA (1990) Auswirkungen des postoperativen Schmerzes auf die Rekonvaleszenz. In: Lehmann KA (ed) Der postoperative Schmerz. Bedeutung, Diagnose und Behandlung. Springer, Berlin p. 96
43. Gürel A, Ünal N, Elevli M, Eren A (1986) Epidural morphine for postoperative pain relief in anorectal surgery. Anesth Analg 65: 499
44. Harmer M, Rosen M, Vickers MD (eds) Patient-controlled analgesia. Blackwell Scientific Publications, Oxford 1985
45. Hashemi K, Middleton MD (1983) Subcutaneous bupivacaine for postoperative analgesia after herniorrhaphy. Ann R Coll Surg Engl 65: 38
46. Heidrich G, Slavic-Svircev V, Kaiko RF (1985) Efficacy and quality of ibuprofen and acetaminophen plus codeine analgesia. Pain 22: 385
47. Henn C, Lehmann KA (1990) Prädiktoren des postoperativen Schmerzes. In: Lehmann KA (ed) Der postoperative Schmerz. Bedeutung, Diagnose und Behandlung. Springer, Berlin: p. 55
48. Hjortso NC, Neumann P, Frosig F, Andersen T, Lindhard A, Rogon E, Kehlet H (1985) A controlled study on the effect of epidural analgesia with local anaesthetics and morphine on morbidity after abdominal surgery. Acta Anaesthesiol Scand 29: 790
49. Hjortso NC, Lund C, Mogensen T, Bigler D, Kehlet H (1986) Epidural morphine improves pain relief and maintains sensory analgesia during continuous bupivacaine after abdominal surgery. Anesth Analg 65: 1033
50. Hunt CO, Naulty JS, Bader AM, Hauch MA, Vartikar JV, Datta S, Hertwig LM, Ostheimer GW (1989) Perioperative analgesia with subarachnoid fentanyl-bupivacaine for caesarean delivery. Anesthesiology 71: 535
51. Jensen MP, Karoly P, Braver S (1986) The measurement of clinical pain intensity: a comparison of six methods. Pain 27: 117
52. Jöhr M (1987) Späte Komplikationen der kontinuierlichen Blockade des N. femoralis. Reg Anaesth 10: 37
53. Jones RM, Cashman JN, Foster JMG, Wedley JR, Adams AP (1985) Comparison of infusions of morphine and lysine acetyl salicylate for the relief of pain following thoracic surgery. Br J Anaesth 57: 259
54. Judkins KC, Harmer M (1982) Haloperidol as an adjunct analgesic in the management of postoperative pain. Anaesthesia 37: 1118
55. Kamban JR, Hammon J, Parris ECV, Lupinetti M (1989) Intrapleural analgesia for postthoracotomy pain and blood levels of bupivacaine following intrapleural injection. Can J Anaesth 36: 106
56. Keats AS (1965) Postoperative pain: research and treatment. J Chronic Dis 4: 72
57. King MJ, Bowden MI, Cooper GM (1990) Epidural fentanyl and 0.5 % bupivacaine for elective caesarean section. Anaesthesia 45: 285
58. Korttila K, Pentti OM, Auvinen J (1980) Comparison of i. m. lysin acetylsalicylate and oxycodone in the treatment of pain after operation. Br J Anaesth 52: 613
59. van Kleef JW, Brum AGL, Vletter AA (1990) Single dose interpleural versus intercostal blockade: nerve block characteristics and plasma concentration profiles after administration of 0.5 % bupivacaine with epinephrine. Anesth Analg 70: 484
60. Lander J (1990) Clinical judgements on pain management. Pain 42: 15
61. Landesberg G, Meretyk S, Lankovsky Z, Shapiro A, Magora F (1990) Intraoperative-intrapleural catheter placement for continuous bupivacaine administration. Eur J Anaesth 7: 149
62. Lanz E, Kehrberger E, Theiss D (1985) Epidural morphine: a clinical double-blind study of dosage. Anesth Analg 64: 786
63. Lehmann KA, Gördes B, Hoeckle W (1985) Postoperative On-Demand Analgesie mit Morphin. Anaesthesist 34: 494
64. Lehmann KA, Henn C (1987) Zur Lage der postoperativen Schmerztherapie in der Bundesrepublik Deutschland. Ergebnisse einer Repräsentativumfrage. Anaesthesist 36: 400

65. Lehmann KA, Heinrich C, van Heiss R (1988) Balanced anaesthesia and patient-controlled postoperative analgesia with fentanyl: minimum effective concentrations, accumulation and acute tolerance. Acta Anaesthesiol Belg 39: 11
66. Lehmann KA, Reichling U,Wirtz R (1988) Influence of naloxone on the postoperative analgesic and respiratory effects of buprenorphine. Eur J Clin Pharmacol 34: 343
67. Lehmann KA (1990) Patient-controlled analgesia for postoperative pain. Adv Pain Res Ther 14: 297
68. Lehmann KA (1990) Der postoperative Schmerz. Bedeutung, Diagnose und Behandlung. Springer, Berlin Heidelberg New York
69. Lehmann KA (1990) Opioide und Antagonisten. Klinische Pharmakologie für Anästhesisten, Intensivmediziner und Schmerztherapeuten. Springer, Berlin Heidelberg New York
70. Lehmann KA (1990) Schmerzmessung und -dokumentation. In: Lehmann KA (ed) Der postoperative Schmerz. Bedeutung, Diagnose und Behandlung. Springer, Berlin Heidelberg New York: p 31
71. Lehmann KA, Gerhard A, Horrichs-Haermeyer G, Zech D (1991) Postoperative patient-controlled analgesia with sufentanil. Analgesic efficacy and minimum effective concentrations. Acta Anaesthesiol Scand: 35: 221
72. Lehmann KA, Kratzenberg U, Schroeder-Bark B, Horrichs-Haermeyer G (1990) Postoperative patient-controlled analgesia with tramadol. Analgesic efficacy and miniumum effective concentrations. Clin J Pain: 6: 212
73. Lehmann KA, Ribbert N, Horrichs-Haermeyer G (1990) Postoperative patient-controlled analgesia with alfentanil. Analgesic efficacy and minimum effective concentrations. J Pain Sympt Manage: 5: 249
74. Levack ID, Holmes JD, Robertson GS (1986) Abdominal wound perfusion for the relief of postoperative pain. Br J Anaesth 58: 615
75. Levine JD, Gordon NC, Smith R, McBryde R (1986) Desipramine enhances opiate postoperative analgesia. Pain 27: 45
76. Lindgren I, Saarnivara L (1985) Comparison of paracetamol and aminophenazone plus diazepam suppositories for anxiety and pain relief after tonsillectomy in children. Acta Anaesthesiol Scand 29: 679
77. Loga WG, El-Baz N, El-Ganzouri A, Cullen M, Staren E, Faber LP, Ivankovich AD (1987) Continuous thoracic epidural analgesia for postoperative pain relief following thoracotomy: a randomized prospective study. Anesthesiology 67: 787
78. London SW (1987) Respiratory depression after single epidural injection of local anesthetic and morphine. Anesth Analg 66: 797
79. Louis C, Freye E, Hartung E, Haag W (1982) Buprenorphin in der periduralen Leitungsanästhesie. Eine vergleichende Untersuchung mit und ohne Bupivacain. Anaesth Intensivther Notfallmed 17: 341
80. Manriquez RG, Pallares V (1978) Continuous brachial plexus block for prolonged sympathectomy and control of pain. Anesth Analg 57: 128
81. Martens M (1982) A significant decrease of narcotic drug usage after orthopaedic surgery. A double-blind study with naproxen. Acta Orthop Belg 48: 900
82. Mather L, Mackie J (1983) The incidence of postoperative pain in children. Pain 15: 271
83. Manuelska EL, Olkkola JT, Korpela R (1988) Does prophylactic intravenous infusion of indomethacin improve the management of postoperative pain in children? Can J Anaesth 35: 123
84. McNicol LR (1986) Lower limb blocks for children. Lateral cutaneous and femoral nerve blocks for postoperative pain relief in paediatric practice. Anaethesia 41: 27
85. McQuay HJ, Caroll D, Moore RA (1988) Postoperative orthopaedic pain – the effect of opiate premedication and local anaesthetic blocks. Pain 33: 291
86. Melzack R, Bentley KC, Jeans ME (1985) Piroxicam versus acetaminophen and placebo for the relief of postoperative dental pain. Curr Ther Res 37: 1134

87. Melzack R, Abbott FV, Zackon W, Mulder DS, Davis MW (1987) Pain on a surgical ward: a survey of the duration and intensity of pain and the effectiveness of medication. Pain 29: 67
88. Miller R, Eisenkraft JB, Cohen M, Toth C, Mora CT, Bernstein JL (1986) Midazolam as an adjunct to meperidine analgesia for postoperative pain. Clin J Pain 2: 37
89. Moss G, Regal ME, Lichtig L (1986) Reducing postoperative pain, narcotics, and length of hospitalization. Surgery 99: 206
90. Mowbray A, Wong KKS, Murray JM (1987) Intercostal catheterization. An alternative approach to the paravertebral space. Anaesthesia 42: 958
91. Murphy DF (1983) Continuous intercostal nerve blockade for pain relief following cholecystectomy. Br J Anaesth 55: 521
92. Naulty JS, Datta S, Ostheimer GW, Johnson MD, Burger GA (1985) Epidural fentanyl for postcaesarean delivery pain management. Anesthesiology 63: 694
93. Neßler R, Schwippel U (1988) Die kontinuierliche Blockade des Plexus lumbalis mit der „3-in-1-Block Kathetertechnik“ in der Schmerztherapie. Reg Anaesth 11: 54
94. Nimmo WS, Todd JG (1985) Fentanyl by constant rate i. v. infusion for postoperative analgesia. Br J Anaesth 57: 250
95. Nuutinen LS, Wuolijoki E, Pentiäinen IT (1986) Diclofenac and oxycodone in treatment of postoperative pain: a double blind trial. Acta Anaesthesiol Scand 30: 620
96. Owen H, Galloway DJ, Mitchell KG (1985) Analgesia by wound infiltration after surgical excision of benign breast lumps. Ann R Coll Surg Engl 67: 114
97. Owen H, Glavin RJ, Shaw NA (1986) Ibuprofen in the management of postoperative pain. Br J Anaesth 58: 1371
98. Owen H, McMillan V, Rogowski D (1990) Postoperative pain therapy: a survey of patients' expectations and their experiences. Pain 41: 303
99. Patel CV, Koppikar MG, Patel MS, Parulkar GB, Pinto Perreira LM (1980) Management of pain after abdominal surgery: dipyrone compared with pethidine. Br J Clin Pharmacol 10: 351S
100. Patel JM, Lanzafame RJ, Williams JS, Mullen BV, Hinshaw JR (1983) The effect of incisional infiltration of bupivacaine hydrochloride upon pulmonary functions, atelectasis and narcotic need following elective cholecystectomy. Surg Gynecol Obstet 157: 228
101. Pryn SJ, Crosse MM, Murison MSC, McGinn FP (1989) Postoperative analgesia for haemorrhoidectomy. A comparison between caudal and local infiltration. Anaesthesia 44: 964
102. Quiding H, Persson G, Ahlström U, Bangens S, Hellem S, Johansson G, Jönsson E, Nordth PG (1982) Paracetamol plus supplementary doses of codeine. An analgesic study of repeated doses. Eur J Clin Pharmacol 23: 315
103. Raj PP, Knarr DC, Vigdorth E, Densson DD, Pither CE, Hartrick CT, Hopson CN, Edström HH (1987) Comparison of continuous epidural infusion of a local anesthetic and administration of systemic narcotics in the management of pain after total knee replacement surgery. Anesth Analg 66: 401
104. Randalls B (1990) Continuous brachial plexus blockade. A technique that uses an axillary catheter to allow successful skin grafting. Anaesthesia 45: 143
105. Ready LB, Oden R, Chadwick HS, Benedetti C, Rooke GA, Caplan R, Wild LM (1988) Development of an anesthesiology-based postoperative pain management service. Anesthesiology 68: 100
106. Reasbeck PG, Rice ML, Reasbeck JC (1982) Double-blind controlled trial of indomethacin as an adjunct to narcotic analgesia after major abdominal surgery. Lancet 2: 115
107. Reiestad F, Stromskag KE (1986) Interpleural catheter in the management of postoperative pain. A preliminary report. Regional Anesthesia 11: 89
108. Rocco A, Reiestad F, Gudman J, McKay W (1987) Intrapleural administration of local anesthetics for pain relief in patients with multiple rib fractures. Preliminary report. Regional Anesthesia 12: 10

109. Rosen M, Absi EG, Webster JA (1985) Suprofen compared to dextropropxyphene hydrochloride and paracetamol (Cosalgesic) after extraction of wisdom teeth under general anaesthesia. Anaesthesia 40: 639
110. Rosenberg PH, Scheinin BMA, Lepäntalo MJA, Lindfors O (1987) Continuous intrapleural infusion of bupivacaine for analgesia after thoracotomy. Anesthesiology 67: 811
111. Rosenblatt R, Pepitone-Rockwell F, McKillop MJ (1979) Continuous axillary analgesia for traumatic hand injury. Anesthesiology 51: 565
112. Rucci FS, Cardamone M, Miglori P (1985) Fentanyl and bupivacaine mixtures for extradural blockade. Br J Anaesth 57: 275
113. Saarnivara L, Metsä-Ketelä T, Männistö P, Vapaatalo H (1980) Pain relief and sputum prostaglandins in adults treated with pethidine, tilidine and indomethacin after tonsillectomy. A double-blind study. Acta Anaesthesiol Scand 24: 79
114. Saarnivara L (1984) Comparison of paracetamol and pentazocine suppositories for pain relief after tonsillectomy in adults. Acta Anaesthesiol Scand 28: 315
115. Safran D, Kahlmann G. Orhant EE, Castelain MH, Journois D (1990) Continuous intercostal blockade with lidocaine after thoracic surgery. Clinical and pharmacokinetic study. Anesth Analg 70: 345
116. Scott LE, Clum GA, Peoples JB (1983) Preoperative predictors of postoperative pain. Pain 15: 283
117. Scheinin B, Asantila R, Orko R (1987) The effect of bupivacaine and morphine on pain and bowel function after colonic surgery. Acta Anaesthesiol Scand 31: 161
118. Seeling W, Lotz P, Schröder M (1984) Lungenfunktion nach abdominellen Eingriffen. Ein Vergleich zwischen kontinuierlicher segmentaler thorakaler Periduralanaesthesie und intramuskulär injiziertem Piritramid. Anaesthesist 33: 408
119. Seeling W, Mayer T, Wörsdorfer O (1985) Postoperative Frühmobilisation des Kniegelenks nach Arthrolyse mit kontinuierlicher Katheterperiduralanaesthesie. Reg Anaesth 8: 1
120. Seeling W, Bruckmooser KP, Hüfner C, Kneitinger E, Rigg C, Rockemann M (1990) Keine Verminderung postoperativer Komplikationen durch Katheterperiduralanalgesie nach großen abdominellen Eingriffen. Anaesthesist 39: 33
121. Seeling W, Kustermann J, Schneider E (1990) Postoperative Katheterperiduralanalgesie nach abdominellen Eingriffen. Bupivacain versus Buprenorphin peridural. Reg Anaesth 13: 78
122. Seltzer JL, Larijani GE, Goldberg ME, Marr AT (1987) Intrapleural bupivacaine – a kinetic and dynamic evaluation. Anesthesiology 67: 798
123. Singh PN, Sharma P, Gupta PK, Pandey K (1981) Clinical evaluation of diazepam for relief of postoperative pain. Br J Anaesth 53: 831
124. Skelbred P, Lokken P (1982) Codeine added to paracetamol induced side effects but did not increase analgesia. Br J Clin Pharmacol 14: 539
125. Sprigge JS, East DSR, Fox GS, Ogilvie RI, Otton PE, Bevan DR (1982) Meperidine infusion for postoperative analgesia in grossly obese patients. Can Anaesth Soc J 29: 142
126. Stenkamp SJ, Easterlin TR, Chadwick HS (1989) Effect of epidural and intrathecal morphine on the length of hospital stay. Anesth Analg 68: 66
127. Tammisto T, Tigerstedt I (1980) Mild analgesics in postoperative pain. Br J Clin Pharmacol 10: 347S
128. Thomas DFM, Lambert WG, Williams KL (1983) The direct perfusion of surgical wounds with local anaesthetic solution: an approach to postoperative pain. Ann R Coll Surg Engl 65: 226
129. Tuominen M, Pitkänen M, Rosenberg PH (1987) Postoperative pain relief and bupivacaine plasma levels during continuous interscalene brachial plexus block. Acta Anaesthesiol Scand 31: 276
130. Tverskov M, Cozacov C, Ayache M, Bradley EL, Kissin I (1990) Postoperative pain after inguinal herniorrhaphy with different types of anesthesia. Anest Analg 70: 29

131. Ullman DA, Fortune RB, Greenhouse BB, Wimpy RE, Kennedy TM (1989) The treatment of patients with multiple rib fractures using continuous epidural narcotic infusion. Regional Anesthesia 14: 43
132. VadeBoncoeur TR, Riegler FX, Gautt RS, Weinberg GL (1989) A randomized, double-blind comparison of the effects of intrapleural bupivacaine and saline on morphine requirements and pulmonary function after cholecystectomy. Anesthesiology 71: 339
133. Valanne J, Korttila K, Ylikorkala O (1987) Intravenous diclofenac sodium decreases prostaglandin synthesis and postoperative symptoms after general anaesthesia in outpatients undergoing dental surgery. Acta Anaesthesiol Scand 31: 722
134. Weis OF, Sriwatanakul K, Alloza JL, Weintraub M, Lasagna L (1983) Attitudes of patients, housestaff, and nurses toward postoperative analgesic care. Anesth Analg 62: 70
135. Winnem B, Samstad B, Breivik H (1981) Paracetamol, tiaramide and placebo for pain relief after orthopaedic surgery. Acta Anaesthesiol Scand 25: 209
136. Wolf AR, Hughes D, Wade A, Mather SJ, Prys-Roberts C (1990) Postoperative analgesia after paediatric orchidopexy: evaluation of a bupivacaine-morphine mixture. Br J Anaesth 64: 430
137. Yamaguchi H, Watanabe S, Motokawa K, Ishizawa Y (1990) Intrathecal morphine dose-response data for pain relief after cholecystectomy. Anesth Analg 70: 168

Cancer Pain

R. PAYNE

Introduction

Cancer pain is an immense problem, as documented by surveys which estimate its prevalence in the developed and developing world. Estimates from the World Health Organization (WHO) [32] demonstrate that up to 25 % of patients worldwide die of unrelieved cancer pain, and as many as 3.5 million people daily experience cancer pain. Survey data from oncological centers in the United States suggest that as many as 60 % of patients in active therapy for cancer experience pain sufficient to reduce their activity, or to require analgesics, and as many as 80 % of patients with advanced cancer have moderate to severe pain [8].

The ability to control cancer pain has improved dramatically in the past several years, and can be related to several factors. Elucidation of ascending and descending neuroanatomical pathways involved in the perception and modulation of nociceptive stimuli has provided a means of understanding pain problems in terms of pathophysiological alterations in the peripheral and central nervous systems. This may potentially allow for more rational and scientifically based therapies [18]. For example, the ability to record neural traffic from single afferent C-nociceptive fibers by the technique of microneurography has allowed the characterization of specific subgroups of neuropathic and sympathetically-maintained pains (the ABC, "angry backfiring C-fiber" syndrome), related to spontaneous and enhanced evoked activity of these nociceptors as a consequence of tissue injury [15]. This may suggest specific new therapies, such as the use of topical agents which selectively affect C-fiber function (i.e., capsaicin) as therapeutic agents in this disorder.

Specific pain syndromes occurring in the cancer patient have been characterized [6], and this may have the effect of suggesting new therapeutic approaches in addition to providing for the early recognition and prompt initiation of specific antitumor and anti-pain therapies. Thus Vecht [29] demonstrated that postmastectomy pain occurring after axillary dissection is caused by injury of the intercostal-brachial radial nerve; therefore the topical application of capsaicin is rational therapy, and indeed has been shown to be possibly effective in relieving pain in one uncontrolled study of this disorder [31].

A major advance in the management of pain in the cancer patient has been an improved understanding of the clinical pharmacology of analgesic drugs, especially opioid analgesics. This includes the delineation of guidelines for appropriate titration of oral morphine and other opioids [20], as well as the use of novel or unconventional routes of opioid administration to enhance their therapeutic ratio [19]. In addition, a new field of clinical pharmacology, which relates the disposition of analgesics in blood and spinal fluid to the intensity of therapeutic and toxic effects (e.g. pharmacokinetic-pharmacodynamic [PK-PD] modelling) has been developed, in part related to evaluation of analgesics in the cancer patient with pain [13].

Finally, psychological factors contributing to the perception of acute and chronic pain, and the related importance of supportive care services which evaluate and attend to the control of psychosocial complications of pain and other symptoms of cancer have received renewed attention [5]. Supportive care services which emphasize the evaluation and treatment of the psychosocial complications of pain enhance the ability to care for cancer patients.

The following discussion will present current important issues in the management of pain in the cancer patient, and will focus on recent innovations in pharmacological therapies of pain in the cancer patient, since drug therapy remains the mainstay treatment of acute and chronic cancer pain. Specifically, the recent evidence supporting the analgesic actions of morphine-6-glucuronide, the role of new modes of drug delivery such as by the transdermal and transmucosal routes of administration, and the controversies inherent in these approaches will be discussed.

Pharmacological Approaches to Cancer Pain Management

Oral Morphine

Oral morphine is the opioid of choice for the management of severe chronic pain in the cancer patient because of its demonstrated efficacy in many studies [32], its linear pharmacokinetics (even in large doses), and the close parallel between its analgesic duration of effect and plasma half-life. Although there is no doubt that oral morphine can be effectively used in cancer pain management, as demonstrated by its substitution for heroin in the Brompton cocktail without loss of efficacy [21], considerable arguments ensue relating to the most accurate determination of its oral/parenteral potency ratio.

Classical single-dose analgesic studies by Houde et al. demonstrated an intramuscular/oral potency ratio of 1:6 [12]. However, Twycross and others suggested that, on the basis of survey data and clinical experience, the intramuscular/oral potency ratio of morphine was 1:2 or 1:3 [28]. This discrepancy may be explained by the recent demonstration of an active metabolite of morphine, morphine-6-glucuronide, which accumulates with repetitive oral and parenteral dosing [17], and has been shown to have analgesic actions in man upon intravenous administration [16]. The 6-glucuronide metabolite of morphine is at least as potent as morphine in animal models of antinociception [10], and its accumulation in blood may well explain the apparent increased potency of oral morphine on repetitive administration, as well as the lack of correlation between plasma morphine concentrations and the time course of clinical effects such as respiratory depression in man [22].

Novel Routes of Administration

In the past several years, newer routes of opioid administration have been utilized in an attempt to more rapidly titrate doses to provide pain relief, or to maintain constant blood or CSF concentrations to minimize side effects and return of pain related to peak and trough oscillations of drug concentrations [19]. The use of patient-controlled analgesia in patients with oral mucositis pain following bone-marrow transplantation is an example where rapid titration of morphine can be undertaken safely, under the patient's control [1]. More recently, transmucosal administration of fentanyl via a lollipop-like "sucker" (known formally as an oral transmucosal unit) [24], the intranasal administration of the agonist-antagonist butorphanol [2], and sublingual administration of buprenorphine [30], provide examples of dosage forms of opioids designed to provide rapid increments in plasma concentrations after even a single administration. On the other hand, spinal, subcutaneous and intravenous infusion, as well as transdermal administration of fentanyl, are examples of modes of drug delivery which aim to provide constant levels of opioid and hence "smoother" pain relief for the cancer patient with continuous chronic pain.

Although many of these routes are in clinical development, their potential usefulness in certain situations is self-evident. For example, movement-induced "incident" or "breakthrough" pain is a common clinical problem for the cancer patient [21], and the ability to rapidly dose a patient in anticipation of movement, or soon after a painful movement, with transnasal, sublingual, or transmucosal dosage forms of an opioid is attractive. The capacity to provide convenient continuous dosing of an opioid such as fentanyl on an outpatient basis for patients with chronic cancer pain in the absence of expensive pumps or needles is likewise appealing. Therefore the pending availability of transdermal fentanyl for the management of cancer pain is an exciting prospect. Further clinical studies defining the relative potency of these opioids with respect to oral morphine, and their efficacy and unique adverse effects relative to conventional opioids and routes of administration, are required.

Controversies in the Pharmacotherapy of Cancer Pain

Two major factors limit physician prescription of opioids for cancer pain management. The first concerns the risks of iatrogenic addiction with chronic administration of opioids. A full discussion of the evidence supporting and refuting significant risks of iatrogenic addiction in the cancer patient is beyond the scope of this chapter, but, in sum, the available data would suggest strongly that the risk of iatrogenic addiction is very small in patients who have not demonstrated a prior history of substance abuse [14]. On the other hand, the rate at which tolerance to opioid actions occurs in the cancer patient is more problematic, and may be dependent on the route of administration. Greenburg [9], Coombs [3] and Cousins [26] demonstrated that rapid dose escalations (and ultimately very large spinal doses) may be required to provide pain relief – and in some instances may even fail to provide pain relief [7] – when morphine is administered by continuous intrathecal infusion to patients with cancer pain, particularly when large systemic doses of opioids were taken prior to the start of spinal infusion.

Furthermore, in the patient with progressive disease, rapid escalations in opioid doses may be required to maintain pain relief [7]. Houde demonstrated a shift in the dose-response curve to the right in patients taking morphine for at least two weeks, indicating that apparent change in receptor sensitivity may occur [12]. But as Twycross has indicated, pharmacological tolerance is seldom an important clinical problem in patients with stable disease [28]. Recently, animal studies have demonstrated that tolerance may be overcome by using opioids with high intrinsic receptor affinity [25], or by alternating drugs with different receptor affinities for μ and δ receptors [23]. This approach has been utilized clinically with the intrathecal administration of D-ala-D-leu[enkephalin] (a relative selective δ agonist which is a structural analogue of leucine enkephalin) to patients rendered tolerant to spinal (or systemic) doses of morphine or hydromorphone (μ agonists) [4].

Conclusions

The investigation of pain in the cancer patient, and particularly its pharmacological management [11], remains at the forefront of clinical activity in oncology. As emphasized in this symposium, new drug delivery systems promise to deliver opioids (and potentially other compounds with analgesic activity) more conveniently and effectively and thus improve their therapeutic ratio. Further clinical research in this area is urgently needed.

References

1. Chapman CR, Hill HF (1989) Prolonged morphine self-administration and addiction liability: evaluation of two theories in a bone marrow transplantation unit. Cancer 63: 1636–1644
2. Cool WM, Kurtz NM, Chu G (1990) Transnasal delivery of systemic drugs. In: Benedetti C, Chapman CR, Giron G (eds) Advances in pain research and therapy. Vol 14. Raven Press, New York pp 241–258
3. Coombs DW, Mauer LH, Saunders RL (1984) Outcomes and complications of continuous intraspinal narcotic analgesia for cancer pain control. J Clin Oncol 2: 1414–1420
4. Coombs DW, Saunders RL, LaChance D, Savage S, Ragnarsson TS, Jensen L (1985) Intrathecal morphine tolerance: use of intrathecal clonidine, DADLE and intraventricular morphine. Anesthesiology 62: 358–363
5. Coyle N (1989) Continuity of care for the cancer patient with chronic pain. Cancer 63: 2289–2293
6. Foley KM (1979) Pain syndromes in patients with cancer. In: Bonica JJ, Ventrafridda V (eds) Advances in pain research and therapy. Vol 2. Raven Press, New York pp 59–75
7. Foley KM (1985) Pharmacological approaches to cancer pain management. In: Fields HL, Dubner R, Cervero F (eds) Advances in pain research and therapy. Vol 9. Raven Press, New York, pp 629–653
8. Foley KM, Arbit E (1989) Management of cancer pain. In: DeVita VT, Hellman S, Rosenberg SA (eds) Cancer: principles and practice of oncology. JB Lippincott, Philadelphia, pp 2064–2087
9. Greenburgh HS, Jaren J, Engminger WD, Doan K (1982) Benefit from and tolerance to continuous intrathecal infusion of morphine in intractable cancer pain. J Neurosurg 57: 360–363
10. Hand CW, Blunnie WP, Claffey LP (1987) Potential analgesic contributions from morphine-6-glucuronide in CSF. Lancet 1: 1207–8
11. Hanks GW (ed) (1988) Cancer surveys: advances and prospects in clinical, epidemiological and laboratory oncology. 7: 1–223
12. Houde RW, Wallenstein SL, Beaver WT (1966) Evaluation of analgesics in patients with cancer pain. In: Lasagna L (ed) International encyclopedia of pharmacology and therapeutics. Section 6. Clinical pharmacology. Pergamon Press, New York, pp 59–99
13. Inturrisi CE, Portenoy RK, Max MB, Colburn WA, Foley KM (1990) Pharmacokinetic-pharmacodynamic relationships of methadone infusions in patients with cancer pain. Clin Pharmacol Ther 47: 565–577
14. Kanner RM, Foley KM (1981) Patterns of narcotic drug use in a cancer pain clinic. Ann NY Acad Sci 362: 162–172
15. Ochoa J (1986) The newly recognized painful ABC syndrome: thermographic aspects. Thermology 2: 99
16. Osborne R, Joel S, Trew D, Slevin M (1988) Analgesic activity of morphine-6-glucuronide. Lancet 1: 828
17. Osborne R, Joel S, Trew D, Slevin M (1990) Morphine and metabolite behavior after different routes of morphine administration: demonstration of the importance of the active metabolite morphine-6-glucuronide. Clin Pharmacol Ther 47: 12–19
18. Payne R (1989) Cancer pain: anatomy, physiology and pharmacology. Cancer 63: 2266–2272
19. Payne R (1989) Novel routes of opioid administration. In: Hill CS, Fields WS (eds) Advances in pain research and therapy. Vol 11. Raven Press, New York pp 319–338
20. Payne R, Max M (1989) Principles of analgesic use in the treatment of acute pain and chronic cancer pain, 2nd ed. American Pain Society, Skokie, Illinois
21. Portenoy R, Hagen NS (1990) Breakthrough pain: definition, prevalence and characteristics. Pain 41: 273–282

22. Rigg JRA (1978) Ventilatory effects and plasma concentration of morphine in man. Br J Anesth 50: 759–65
23. Russel RD, Chang KJ (1989) Alternated delta and mu receptor activation: a strategem for limiting opioid tolerance. Pain 36: 381–389
24. Stanley TH, Hague B, Mock DL, Streisand JB, Bubbers S, Dzelzkalns RR, Bailey PL, Pace NL, East KA, Ashburn MA (1989) Oral transmucosal fentanyl citrate (lollipop) premedication in human volunteers. Anesth Analg 69: 21–27
25. Stevens CW, Yaksh TL (1989) Potency of infused spinal antinociceptive agents is inversely related to magnitude of tolerance after continuous infusion. J Pharm Exp Ther 250: 1–8
26. Tanetian DL, Cousins LM (1990) Failure of massive doses of spinal morphine to control cancer pain in a patient previously treated with systemic morphine. Pain 36: 359–362
27. Twycross RG (1977) Choice of strong analgesic in terminal cancer: diamorphine or morphine? Pain 3: 93–104
28. Twycross RW, Lack SA (1983) Symptom control in far advanced cancer: pain relief. Pitman, London
29. Vecht CJ, van Debrand HJ, Wajer OJM (1989) Post-axillary dissection pain in breast cancer due to a lesion of the intercostobrachial nerve. Pain 36: 171–176
30. Vincenti E (1990) Sublingual opiates in acute pain. In: Benedetti C, Chapman CR, Giron S (eds) Advances in pain research and therapy. Vol 14. Raven Press, New York pp 227–231
31. Watson CP, Evans RJ, Watt VR (1989) The postmastectomy pain syndrome and the effect of topical capsaicin. Pain 38: 177–186
32. World Health Organisation (1986). Cancer pain relief. Geneva

Pain Management and Quality of Life in Cancer Patients

C. M. MOINPOUR and C. R. CHAPMAN

Introduction

Because of advances in early diagnosis and treatment, more patients are surviving cancer, and many who ultimately succumb do so only after a period of significantly extended life. Unfortunately, many patients pay a high price for effective treatment. Both the neoplasm and the cytodestructive interventions directed at it degrade the well-being of the cancer patient, and some patients who survive cancer suffer reduced functional capability, chronic symptom problems, and/or persisting pain. Consequently, patient comfort and function during extended life and survival are emerging as pressing concerns in cancer care [91].

Pain control is a critical element in the comprehensive care of many cancer patients. Multiple painful diagnostic and therapeutic events and pain problems occur in the long interval between disease diagnosis and termination of treatment, and many terminally ill patients experience severe pain in the last weeks or days of life. Unremitting pain overshadows every other aspect of human existence, destroys hope and courage, and brings the family as well as the patient to the brink of desperation. Consequently, we urgently need definitive research in this area [12].

Evaluation of therapeutic outcome trials for pain control in cancer patients may well be the greatest challenge in clinical pain research. Most cancer patients have multiple pain problems over long time periods. Moreover, researchers limited to standard unidimensional pain or pain relief rating tools cannot address the overarching question of how pervasively persisting pain degrades life. Comprehensive evaluation of patient well-being requires multidimensional evaluation with multiple therapeutic endpoints. The emergence of new theory and tools for the study of Quality of Life (QOL) in cancer patients suggests new horizons for therapeutic outcome trials in the cancer pain field.

In this chapter we examine the problem of cancer-related pain and explore the possibility of studying pain relief in terms of QOL. We then review related progress and issues in the QOL research area, providing overviews of several useful conceptual frameworks and assessment methods. We discuss ways in which QOL research could contribute to the comprehensive evaluation of pain management strategies and offer suggestions for developing studies in this area. Finally, we formulate conclusions about the value of QOL research strategies and tools for the study of therapeutic outcome in cancer pain research.

Pain and Cancer

The nature of cancer pain is the basic groundwork for discussion of research on pain control. Pain in patients with cancer is neither singular nor constant. It accompanies both disease and treatment, changes over time, and multiple pain problems can exist simultaneously [113]. Pain as an aversive sensation interacts with the emotional state of the patient and affects the patient's cognitions to produce a complex pattern of suffering. Considered broadly, pain degrades life. In this section we review the scope of cancer pain as a medical problem and briefly review the mechanisms that produce cancer-related pain; finally, we discuss the related concept of suffering.

Magnitude of the Problem

Recent estimates indicate that cancer pain relief is a pressing global problem. Bonica [12] drew upon data in 54 reports from 15 countries and estimated that, in 1986, 8.8 million persons worldwide experienced pain associated with cancer. Recognizing that pain depends on the type and site of tumor present, he projected that 20%–50% of patients have pain at the time of diagnosis and that 55%–95% have pain when the disease is far advanced, with an overall average approaching 75%. Roughly 40%–50% of those with advanced cancer have moderate to severe pain, and another 25%–30% suffer very severe or excruciating pain. After examining a subset of reports drawn from cancer centers and hospitals, Bonica concluded that 75%–80% of patients in terminal stage, or who have far advanced disease, require opioid therapy for pain.

As Twycross and Fairfield [112] demonstrated, most cancer patients with pain have multiple pain problems. Several studies in the United States by Foley and colleagues [27, 38, 59] suggest that tumor causes the dominant pain problem in about three quarters of patients, and cancer treatment complications or toxicities produce most of the remainder. Fortunately, 80%–90% of cancer-related pain can be controlled by drugs administered in accordance with WHO guidelines [107].

Since the likelihood of persons in industrialized countries dying of other causes has been decreasing steadily, many will contract cancer at an advanced age. The incidence of cancer deaths is therefore unlikely to drop in the foreseeable future, despite modest progress in early diagnosis and treatment [95]. Moreover, ever more aggressive treatments tend to produce more survivors with more painful complications. The scope of the problem of cancer pain in developed countries may well increase in coming decades unless major breakthroughs in the prevention and cure of cancer emerge.

Mechanisms of Pain

Basic Mechanisms

Pain can originate with nociception, i.e., the activation of small unmyelinated or thinly myelinated sensory nerve endings that detect and signal tissue damage or threat to tissue [118]. Nociception is heightened when inflammation is present since inflammatory processes produce or release chemicals that sensitize nociceptors and produce hyperalgesia (prostaglandins, bradykinin, substance P).

Neuropathic mechanisms can also produce pain. Compression of a nerve or direct injury to a nerve or its myelin sheath can cause abnormal firing patterns that produce paresthesia or pain, even when the nociceptive field of the nerve is uninjured. Partial or total destruction of a peripheral nerve or plexus or of spinal cord or brain stem pathways can cause deafferentation pain [12]. Some nociceptive and neuropathic conditions occur as a consequence of disorders of immune function. Disease processes and treatment complications activate one or more of these mechanisms to produce pain.

Disease Processes

Tumors can generate pain by infiltration of sensitive structures such as bone, nerve or plexus, or solid viscus, through obstruction of hollow viscus, vein or artery, by compression of spinal cord or other neural structures, and via production of inflammatory response [12, 89]. Most cancer pain originates in primary or metastatic bone tumors, and invasion of neurologic structures is the second most common cause [12].

Tumor invasion of bone occurs frequently with lung and hormone-dependent tumors. It commonly involves vertebral body metastases that produce back and neck pain, base of skull metastases that cause head and face pain, and pelvic or long bone pain. Epidural spinal cord compression can occur with pain, following radicular patterns.

Invasion of plexuses, nerve roots, or spinal cord can be exquisitely painful. Vertebral fracture secondary to bone metastasis can cause sudden nerve or nerve root compression. Tumor invasion of neural structures results in constant neuralgia with a burning quality. When tumor encroaches on the lumbosacral plexus or brachial plexus, pain manifests in radiculopathic or other neurologic patterns.

Obstruction of hollow visceral organs by tumor results in intense smooth muscle contraction, producing diffuse and often referred pain. Ulceration and hemorrhage in visceral structures also cause pain. Tumor-induced necrosis can contribute to pancreatic pain.

Infiltration of blood vessels, or occlusion of a blood vessel, by tumor may produce ischemia or venous engorgement with consequent edema. The superior vena caval syndrome distends neck veins and produces facial edema, often with chest pain and headache.

Treatment-Related Pain Mechanisms

Pain problems associated with antineoplastic treatment are both acute and chronic. Most patients experience repeated treatment-related pain problems between diagnosis of cancer and termination of treatment. We identify four types of treatment-related pain: (a) procedure-related acute pain, (b) toxicity-related acute and chronic pain, (c) acute and chronic pain resulting from surgical iatrogenesis, and (d) acute and chronic pain associated with other complications. Multiple mechanisms contribute to these complex problems.

Pain can occur as a result of both diagnostic and therapeutic procedures that activate nociceptors. Common painful diagnostic procedures include bone marrow aspiration, biopsy, endoscopy, and angiography [22]. Some therapeutic procedures, including those often performed for palliation, such as tumor embolization, are markedly painful [100], as are complications such as extraversion of a chemotherapeutic drug.

Neuropathic mechanisms, nociception and inflammation are often at work simultaneously in toxicity. Chemotherapy toxicities include arthralgias and myalgias, painful peripheral neuropathies, organ injury such as acute pancreatitis, and severe oral mucositis [55, 103]. Painful acute conditions can follow radiation such as oropharyngeal inflammation and mucosal ulceration [85]. Neuropathies also occur. Transient and progressive postradiation myelopathy, peripheral nerve tumors, and late onset fibrosis of the brachial or lumbar plexus are all painful radiation toxicities.

Cancer surgeries cause acute and sometimes chronic postoperative pain, including intractable deafferentation pain, via nociceptive, inflammatory and neuropathic mechanisms. Several iatrogenic cancer surgery pain syndromes are well known [12]. Damage to the intercostobrachial nerve during radical mastectomy can cause delayed onset pain in the arm and axilla, which typically emerges 4–8 weeks post-surgery. Radical neck dissection sometimes produces chronic burning and lancinating pain accompanied by dysesthesias. Phantom limb pain occurs in some patients following surgical amputation.

Other painful complications include microbial infection in immune suppressed individuals [92], symptoms of graft-versus-host disease following bone marrow transplantation [10, 92], and the diffuse arthralgias and myalgias of steroid pseudorheumatism, a condition observed in patients withdrawn from steroids [94].

The incidence, severity and duration of such problems are still ill defined for cancer patients with frequently occurring diseases such as lung, breast, and prostate cancer. Consequently, we can only conjecture that the distress of recurring pains, more often unrelieved than not, and the prospect of more painful episodes in the future, wear down the courage of patients and their families. Twycross and Lack [113] described a vicious circle of "insomnia-fatigue-pain-insomnia" that exhausts and demoralizes patients. Nurses and other health care professionals who work closely with cancer patients commonly observe that treatment-related pain problems severely distress and discourage many, causing some to abandon potentially life-saving therapy. In addition, such pains can mask the recurrence of tumor and delay timely intervention.

Cancer Pain and Suffering

The psychological toll of cancer is high: patients relentlessly face impending death, unrelieved aversive symptoms, loss of functional capability and associated vocational and family roles, frustration, and uncertainty about the future. Pain, when present, is often the focus of patient suffering, and pain complaint often becomes a language vehicle by which the patient can express his global misery.

Medicine has done little to specifically prevent or alleviate suffering, perhaps because the concept is abstract and inconsistently defined. Some rigorous medical researchers reject the term outright as a lay concept. Fortunately, suffering has attracted the attention of many clinicians and researchers in recent years, and useful definitions of suffering are emerging.

Cassell defined human suffering as any perceived threat to the integrity of the individual, where integrity encompasses the psychosocial and psychological, as well as the biological, aspects of the person [17, 18]. He emphasized that suffering is a condition of persons (as opposed to organisms) intrinsically linked to the personhood of the individual. Portenoy [91] described suffering as a global aversive experience that is sustained over time by multiple aversive negative perceptions including (but not limited to) pain. Portenoy's definition emphasizes that suffering in cancer patients is not a static state but rather a dynamic process spanning a window of time and encompassing many catastrophic events.

However we formally define it, suffering is an enduring state that occurs in response to a chronic or prolonged intensively stressful situation, often with many stressors. Pain from metastatic disease may be a prominent cause of a cancer patient's suffering, but one must look at the whole person over time – personal losses, surgical mutilation, inability to cope with repeated procedural distress or pain, social separation during inpatient stay, etc. – to understand his suffering, even when the disease causes severe pain. Suffering differs from fear in that the latter term is limited to event-specific or situation-specific alarm reactions commonly associated with negative expectation.

Suffering often has multiple sustaining determinants that exist in a complex network of cause-and-effect relationships. For example, severe pain impairs human relationships, blocks treasured recreational pursuits, and damages the self-image of normally active, productive persons. These losses foster depression, and this in turn impairs sleep and exacerbates fatigue. Trapped in the vicious circle of pain and insomnia, patients become increasingly negative, withdrawn, and dysphoric.

Compassionate care of the cancer patient requires that caregivers assess and address suffering or use some conceptual scheme that encompasses suffering. It is not enough to attend to isolated symptoms with pharmacologic, surgical or other technical solutions. Clearly, caregivers treating cancer patients must work with well conceptualized, measurable therapeutic endpoints that represent comprehensive care if they are to prevent or relieve suffering.

Toward a Comprehensive Pain and QOL Assessment Model

We suggest that one can approach palliative therapeutic outcome issues such as pain management and more broadly, suffering, via a QOL framework. We also maintain that a reasonable armory of well-refined QOL assessment measures exists. Here we provide a foundation for this approach, discussing key concepts and definitions and addressing basic measurement issues.

Patient Report

Physicians and other health care providers commonly judge and record the functional capability or well-being of cancer patients. Such procedures, which sometimes involve family member judgments, are termed proxy reports. Examples of commonly used physician-rated scales are: the Karnofsky performance status (KPS) scale [58]; the shorter version of the KPS endorsed by the World Health Organization (WHO) and known variously as the ECOG (Eastern Cooperative Oncology Group), Zubrod, or WHO performance status scale [19, 99, 120, 123]; physician-rated toxicities scales used in cooperative group trials; and the Spitzer QL-Index, a brief index of five dimensions of QOL that can be completed by physicians, other health professionals, and patients [104]. However, the literature indicates poor agreement between proxy and patient reports both for physician proxies [13, 64, 65, 81, 102, 117] and for family member/spouse proxies [25, 63, 102]. Consequently, we advocate assessing pain and its impact on patient QOL via *patient* report, as does the International Association for the Study of Pain [53].

Although we emphasize patient report, physician (or other proxy) measures of patient pain and QOL are still useful. Proxy measures can provide additional perspectives on patient functioning as long as patient report provides the primary endpoint for treatment evaluation. Researchers can collect proxy report throughout a study assessment period with the goals of (a) estimating the agreement between patient and proxy report, and (b) knowing the extent of agreement, substituting a proxy measure for patient report in cases where the patient is too ill to comply with data collection requirements.

Self report methods require particular care for very young and very sick patients, but most problems are surmountable. Child report of pain can yield valid and reliable measures [11]. A number of references describe current approaches for obtaining child report of pain [54, 70, 71, 76, 88, 93, 114]. Detailed description of child assessment techniques exceeds the scope of this chapter. We also refrain from discussing the special problems associated with management of pain in elderly patients as, for example, the effect of dementia, particularly of the Alzheimer type, and other syndromes in the elderly such as sleep disturbance on pain report [49]. Harkins et al. [49] note the greater potential for social and emotional disruption within this group of patients.

Definitions of QOL For Cancer Pain Research

Constraints

We address here definitions and assessment methods suitable for a cancer research setting and useful for studies of pain relief. We are concerned with those aspects of a patient's life most likely to be degraded by pain and safeguarded by a pain management intervention. We exclude those broader aspects of the quality of a person's life unlikely to be affected by pain or its relief but historically included by others as indicators of general QOL such as satisfaction with occupation, housing, etc. [8, 15]. The term health-related QOL [56, 86, 87] reflects our restricted definition of QOL.

Use of a QOL vs Suffering Framework

Portenoy [91] suggested that suffering can be defined as impaired QOL. He argued that the lack of a data base relating pain to suffering renders the suffering concept problematic in a research setting. Use of a QOL framework and existing QOL assessment mechanisms can not only address the broad impact of pain (and its relief through intervention) on a patient's life but also provide a more credible assessment methodology.

Lee and Rowlingston [60] argued that persistent pain degrades a patient's lifestyle to such an extent that, from the patient's perspective, his/her QOL deteriorates. They advocated measuring

1. sensory experiences (i.e., intensity, frequency, duration, and location of pain along with comparisons to other pain situations);
2. affective or emotional states (i.e., associated distress or suffering produced by the effect of pain on patient well-being); and
3. behavioral consequences of experiencing pain (e.g., effect on functional and role status resulting in dependence on others, medication use, etc.)

Whether an investigator selects a suffering or QOL rubric, he/she must use a multidimensional conceptualization of the broader impacts of pain and its treatment on the patient. This is because reports of pain intensity/frequency and pain relief following some pain relief intervention insufficiently describe the degree to which pain interferes with a patient's normal functioning and the degree to which different pain treatments restore such functioning.

Impact of Disease: WHO Perspective

The WHO [119] has defined health multidimensionally: "Health is not only the absence of infirmity and disease but also a state of physical, mental and social well-being". Cancer patients experiencing pain identified the same three aspects of QOL as salient: physical well-being; psychological well-being; social/role functioning [84].

More recently, WHO [71, 121] characterized the impact of disease on individuals at the level of a) the *occurrence* of a disease or disorder, b) an *impairment* experienced through symptoms; a *disability* as it affects ability to carry out activities of daily living and c) a *handicap* when the consequences affect the social realm of the person's life with potential for social disadvantages and discrimination.

This perspective can encompass pain as a symptom of cancer or a complication of its treatment and is consistent with QOL approaches to patient assessment. WHO has identified cancer pain as a major international problem [107].

Rationale for Multidimensional QOL Assessment Models

Most health status and QOL measures address at least the three dimensions of health identified by WHO. Shumaker et al. [101] asserted that a multidimensional assessment approach is particularly important when we know little about the effects of the disease and/or treatment of the disease on the individual. Ware [116] advocated casting the widest possible net in early attempts at evaluating the effect of medical interventions on patient QOL. The models of pain assessment identified above similarly emphasize the potential breadth of the impact of severe or chronic pain on a person's life. The belief that a pain assessment model requires description of multiple dimensions of the patient's life space or QOL conforms to the multidimensional assessments of QOL currently used in other clinical trials research. Strang and Qvarner [108] found that intensity of cancer-related pain was related to report of anxiety and depression and to disruption in the areas of physical and social functioning. Tannock et al. [110] found that improvement in multiple areas of QOL and in well-being coincided with reduction in pain associated with bone metastases from prostate cancer.

Representative Multidimensional Models

There are many conceptual schemes for assessing QOL. Most have been designed to assess the impact of a disease on the patient; none are specifically developed for pain research. However, the dimensions identified in several schemes seem well suited for use in studies of pain control in cancer patients. We limit our review here to such instruments.

Cella and Tulsky [20] described ten frequently assessed dimensions in QOL research with cancer patients: functional ability (activity), occupational functioning, social functioning, emotional well-being, family well-being, spirituality, future orientation (planning, hope), sexuality/intimacy (including body image), and physical concerns (symptoms, pain). Cella and Tulsky [20] argued that a multidimensional measure requires inclusion of at least three of these dimensions. Schipper [98] considered the four dimensions of somatic sensation, psychological functioning, social functioning, and physical and occupational functioning as key domains of QOL. Ferrans [40] measures health and functioning, socioeconomic, psychological/spiritual, and family dimensions.

Ware and his colleagues [105, 106, 115] developed instruments to assess six components of overall health and wellness: physical functioning, role functioning, social functioning, mental health, health perceptions, and pain.

The European Organization for Research and Treatment of Cancer (EORTC) QOL study group has included measures of seven *core* dimensions in their QOL instrument (currently under development): functional status, physical symptoms, psychological distress, social interaction, financial/economic impact, perceived health status, and overall QOL [1, 4]. The EORTC approach also allows for *modules* specific to the disease site of interest. Aaronson [3] reported consensus on the importance of measuring four QOL domains: functional status, disease-related and treatment-related symptoms, psychological functioning, and social functioning.

Most QOL assessment models include patient report of global or overall QOL, often as a single-item measure. One can argue that global QOL is not a pure dimension but that it cuts across the primary dimensions variously specified by individual research teams. Consensus exists that a global measure allows patients to summarize treatment experiences and that it adds information about patients' experiences not tapped by the domain-specific measures [80]. These concerns point to pressing problems of measurement in the QOL area.

Measurement Issues

QOL researchers concerned with the sickness impact of specific diseases struggle with the types of problems outlined in the following sections. These issues are relevant to pain management research and so we briefly review them here.

Generic vs Disease-Specific Assessment Approaches

The distinction between generic and disease-specific measures raises issues for the development of multidimensional pain assessment models [86]. Generic health status or QOL measures are those that are broad-based, addressing the effect of the disease and/or treatment on normal, everyday functioning. The items reflect no specific disease- or treatment approach. Disease-specific measurement items are tailored to the disease (e.g., cancer or arthritis) and/or treatment (e.g., chemotherapy), either through reference to the disease or treatment in the wording of items or by selection of items that target a particular disease or treatment. Obviously, researchers can use generic measures in most treatment contexts and can therefore compare the QOL of patients with a variety of medical problems or the effect of several different treatments on the same disease. Generic pain assessment measures appeal because pain is a major symptom associated with a number of diseases and treatments.

Core Plus Module

This approach includes a core set of items covering more generic aspects of QOL with a set of items (module) specific to the disease or treatment of interest in the trial; more than one module could be needed. The EORTC QOL questionnaire [1, 4, 5] is an example of the core plus module approach used in cancer clinical trials. A recent American example is the Southwest Oncology Group QOL questionnaire [75, 77]. A core plus module framework could guide the development of pain assessment instruments as well. The module would contain a very disease-specific set of pain items, while more generic measures could address the broader impacts of pain described above in the Portenoy [91] and Lee and Rowlingson [60] models.

Single Instruments vs a Battery of Measures

Finally, pain researchers can choose between a single instrument with subscales assessing the multiple dimensions of pain versus a set of separate measures, each of which addresses a key dimension of interest. Depending on the number of dimensions in his/her pain assessment model, the researcher is unlikely to find a single instrument that adequately addresses all of the generic dimensions and also comprehensively assesses pain. We present examples of both approaches below.

Psychometric Properties

Any pain or QOL measure must possess adequate psychometric properties. The key properties for pain assessment research are reliability, validity, and sensitivity or responsiveness to change.

Reliability refers to the consistency with which an instrument measures a QOL dimension. If the instrument assesses a single dimension, internal consistency techniques provide a good estimate of instrument reliability [28]. When the instrument covers multiple dimensions and produces a total score, internal consistency may not be appropriate and the researcher should use other techniques such as test–retest reliability [82].

An instrument is valid if it measures what it purports to measure: content, criterion, and construct validity techniques assess this property [6, 16, 82].

Particularly if we evaluate a pain management strategy, we must be able to detect change in reported pain and patient QOL. Because of the time required to demonstrate an instrument's responsiveness, we have less information about this property for established QOL and pain instruments. There are many ways to document an instrument's sensitivity to change [36, 47, 48].

We recommend selecting measures of pain and QOL that have published evidence of adequate psychometric properties. This means minimizing the development of new measures since the establishment of an instrument's psychometric properties requires an enormous investment of time and resources. One can choose existing measures for the more generic dimensions of QOL. The Core Plus Module approach often requires the investigator to develop the disease-specific module. Some research groups such as the Southwest Oncology Group rely on the clinical experience of physician/nurse investigators to identify relevant content for disease- and treatment-specific symptom scales. Psychometric properties, particularly reliability, are ascertained for this set of items after trial data have been obtained.

In addition to reporting existing psychometric data for an instrument, pain researchers should always report reliabilities obtained for these scales with the group of patients they assessed. We recommend small-scale pilot studies to confirm that items (both generic and disease-/treatment-specific) are relevant to the patient population of interest in the research.

Attribution of Effect

Requiring the patient to ascribe his pain to a source or to identify the cause of degraded normal functioning can be perilous. Stewart [106] reported the frequency of comorbid conditions among patients with chronic diseases. The presence of other conditions makes it very difficult for a patient to isolate the exact cause of a symptom's impact on QOL. Patients also have trouble distinguishing the effect of the disease from that of coexisting treatment toxicity or complications on overall functioning. Moreover, some patients are better at self-report than others, and individual differences in self-judgment ability contribute to measurement error. We recommend directing patients to report the existence or occurrence of a problem or limitation whether or not they can directly attribute it to the intervention or disease of interest. By collecting additional information on comorbid conditions, researchers may be able to adjust patients' reports of pain and QOL by taking into account confounding influences.

Value Attached to Health State

Few QOL and pain assessment instruments quantify the degree to which a patient considers a symptom or limitation important (i.e., the degree to which the patient is willing to "live with" the condition). Some researchers have weighted reported symptoms and QOL impacts according to the preference patients indicate for various health states to produce quality adjusted life years (QALYs) [57, 111] or time without symptoms of disease and treatment (TWiST) [46]. Usually these approaches require more complex data collection procedures to obtain utility functions. Some instruments currently under development include a report of health and QOL problems along with the patient's assessment of how important a given problem is to him or her [41]. Consideration of patient valuing of health states and methods for both obtaining and incorporating such values into the QOL assessment model remain ongoing methodologic problems.

Examples of Suitable QOL Instruments

Table 1 lists plausible instruments for assessing multidimensional aspects of the pain experience for patients with life-threatening disease. These instruments all possess adequate psychometric properties (e.g., reliability estimates of at least .7; some evidence of validity). The table depicts the number of items in each instrument, the number of items devoted to pain if it is a more generic instrument, the number (and nature) of QOL dimensions addressed, and key citations for further information. We stress that the instruments in Table 1 are only suggestions. The list is incomplete and these instrument come from a larger pool of possible measures. Many excellent reviews of QOL measures exist [e.g., see 2, 9, 19, 20, 24, 30, 33, 37, 39, 43, 51, 75, 79, 99].

In Table 1, we first list instruments developed to assess pain. The list excludes single-item measures. Chapman and Syrjala [23] noted that single dimension reports of pain typically take one of three forms: verbal descriptor scales such as the Melzack [74] pain intensity scale ("none, mild, discomforting, distressing, horrible, excruciating"), numeric rating scales (e.g., one to ten scale), and visual analogue scale/linear analogue scale assessment (VAS/LASA), which uses a 10-cm line with verbal anchors at each end. The VAS approach requires special training so that patients understand the role of the anchor statements and how they are to mark the line. For further considerations see the chart prepared by Chapman and Syrjala [23] for instrument selection strategies depending on the type of pain expected (e.g., brief acute pain vs acute persistent pain).

In summary, we recommend that researchers identify key QOL dimensions relevant to their pain management research question and select measures that assess those dimensions. As a single instrument will rarely cover all needed dimensions, a battery approach is often appropriate. Many of the suggested instruments are brief and quick to administer. When in doubt, it is better to "cast the broader net", as suggested by Ware [116].

Table 1. Instruments for assessing multidimensional aspects of pain

Instrument Name	No. Items	No. pain Items	Dimensions
True generic:			
Medical outcome study short Form – 36 (MOS-36) [105, 106]	36	2	PI, PRF PhF, RF, EmotF, SocF, HPer
McMaster health index questionnaire (MHIQ)[21]	59–69	0	PhF/RF, EmotF, SocF
Nottingham health profile (Part I)[52]	38	8	a PhF, RF, EmotF, SocF, Fat,
Generic-Cancer:			
EORTC quality of life Questionnaire [1, 4]	36	1	PA, PhF, RF, EmotF, SocF, Fat Sym, Fin, Global
Cancer rehabilitation evaluation system-research version [44, 50, 96, 97]	9	1	PA, PhF, RF, EmotF, SocF, IS/Fam, MI, Global (Total Score)
Generic-arthritis:			Multi Pain Domains
Arthritis impact measurement scale (AIMS) [62, 72]	48/67	4	PhF, EmotF
Generic/domain-specific: pain	17	same	Multi pain intensity domains (Sensory, Affective), Total Score
McGill pain questionnaire (MPQ) short vers. [73, 74, 78]			
Memorial pain assessment card (MPAC) [42]	4	3	Multi pain domains EmotF (mood)
Brief pain inventory (BPI) [26, 29]			Multi pain domains PhF, SocF, EmotF (specific to pain)
Generic/domain-specific: psychosocial	46	0	PhF, RF, SocF, EmotF, Fam, IS, HCO, Global (Total Score)
Psychosocial adjustment to illness scale-self report (PAIS-SR)[34, 35]			
Generic/domain-specific: symptoms	13	2	PF, PI Sym, Out
symptom distress scale [66–69, 122]			
Rotterdam symptom checklist (RSCL)[31, 32]	42/43	6	PI (e.g., muscle, eye, mouth soreness, back pain) PhF, RF, EmotF, Sym, Global
Disease-specific: breast cancer	30	2	PA, PF PhF, EmotF, SocF, Fat, Sym
Breast cancer chemotherapy questionnaire (BCCQ)[61]			

PI = pain intensity; PA = pain amount; PF = pain frequency; PRF = Effect of pain on role functioning; EmotF = emotional functioning; PhF = physical functioning; RF = role functioning; SocF = social functioning; HPer = health perceptions; Sym = symptoms; Fam = family well-being; Fin = financial difficulties; IS = intimacy/sexuality; HCO = health care orientation; Out = outlook; Fat = fatigue/energy; MI = interaction with medical system; a pain items answered by yes or no but weighted on terms of perceivel severity

Design and Analysis Issues in Controlled Clinical Trials

Design Issues

Sampling

Investigators do well to avoid convenience samples and to employ a careful sampling strategy (e.g., every fifth patient). Sample size requirements are not arbitrary but rather follow from power estimation exercises. Investigators should identify several key endpoints among the many components and estimate treatment arm effects with respect to pain reduction and other QOL measures. This process is easiest for symptom measures. It becomes progressively harder as the QOL component becomes more abstract (e.g.,with emotional functioning and global QOL).

Patient inclusion and exclusion criteria are essential. Questionnaires require a certain level of patient literacy. Often researchers state exclusion criteria in terms of ability to complete the questionnaire; that is, mental competence and absence of psychiatric disturbances that could impair ability to complete the questionnaire.

Language ability is also a major consideration. Many QOL questionnaires exist only in one language. Unless an investigator has a carefully translated and written version of the QOL questionnaire (or interview) in the appropriate language, he or she must exclude patients who do not speak that language. Careful translations usually involve forward (i.e., into a second language) and backward (i.e., back into the original language) transcriptions because of the difficulty inherent in capturing QOL concepts. For example, emotional functioning and global QOL are not easily translated and carry cultural meanings in addition to the different words used to express these ideas. It is unacceptable to do on-the-spot translations with local translators at the clinical center. If patients speaking a single language are included in the trial, results can be generalized only to this group.

Minimizing loss-to-follow-up is a key concern in producing a patient sample free from bias. This is a particularly difficult problem in multicenter trials. Investigators must establish a number of quality control procedures to enhance data collection over time. We recommend having a QOL contact person at each major assessment site, training these individuals in the importance of maintaining compliance with longitudinal data collection, and preparing calendars and other reminders for data collectors.

Timing of Assessments

One of the more difficult design problems is identifying meaningful times for assessment so that pain interventions (or treatments that reduce tumor size or achieve palliation in other ways) can be "fairly" compared. Knowledge of the natural course of the disease and its effect on increasing or decreasing pain is crucial in determining when to measure QOL. If the investigator compares two pain treatments that differ in expected time to pain relief or in the timing of the regimen, this complicates the timing of QOL assessments. Generally, daily diaries are the most thorough method for tracking treatment effects and providing QOL profiles over time (e.g., see [45]). However, daily data collection (even if they are brief four-or-five-item measures, which we do not recommend) is often impractical in multicenter settings. In such cases, we recommend assessing all patients at the same calendar time points even though that might result in more assessments if key points differ for the treatment arms.

There are many potential pitfalls in repeated clinical assessments that investigators do well to forecast before beginning a study. In trials comparing treatments that affect tumor (whether curative or palliative), it is important to continue assessing patient QOL if one regimen's course is completed while the other is ongoing. Other problems for interpretation occur if assessments stop when a patient is asymptomatic and elects to stop treatment, the disease recurs, and the patient begins another treatment, or the patient experiences some problem with one of the treatments. Careful follow-up is essential in order to detect long-term effects of a treatment. Investigators must decide whether to measure patients just before treatment occurs or immediately or shortly after (if acute toxic effects of the treatment are of interest).

Analysis Issues

Multivariate Correlated Outcomes

Once an investigator decides upon a multidimensional definition for QOL, he or she faces a "multiple endpoints" problem. This hurdle is hardly new. Clinical trials research often involves multiple endpoints; for example, in cancer clinical trials, investigators examine survival, disease-free survival, time to relapse, tumor size, etc. Similarly, in pain research one might have: worse pain for the day, least pain for the day, number of incidences of "breakthrough pain", pain relief, etc.

Fortunately, there are several ways to deal with multiple endpoints. First, investigators can identify in advance the key components for statistical comparisons between patient groups and then relegate other QOL components to the level of exploratory analyses. Southwest Oncology Group QOL studies use this approach: physical and emotional functioning and three symptoms are examined at three time points. Investigators adjust the criterion for statistical significance (alpha), typically dividing alpha = .05 by 15 comparisons; this is, admittedly, a conservative approach. This method holds the multiple testing problem at bay until statistical techniques "catch up" to the problem. Some alternatives already exist [90].

A second straightforward approach is to plot multiple QOL endpoints at single time points by treatment arm. Likewise, one can compare plots of single QOL components over time. It is always reasonable to plot individual curves for patients in order to examine the degree of variability present among patients over time. This facilitates the interpretation of group trends. For example, average report of pain intensity or pain relief over groups of patients may or may not represent the typical patient, depending on the degree of variability present within a group.

If sample size is sufficient and loss to follow-up is minimal, investigators can use "repeated measures" approaches for those endpoints, targeting total scores. One can opt for overlapping repeated measures techniques when dropout over time has been more substantial than expected. It is useful to determine whether, as the sample decreases over time, patients in and out of the sample differ on important variables. For example, with patients in the data base for assessment one, investigators can compare differences on key prognostic and predictor variables between those who did and those who did not provide data for assessment two. One can similarly compare sample differences at all time points. Nonrandom missing data (e.g., from patients too sick to complete questionnaires) pose the worst problem for analysis. However, Brown [14] suggests ways of handling even these types of data.

Weighting and Combining QOL Components

Investigators sometimes wish to combine pain measures and QOL components into some more global index reflecting the effect of the pain management intervention. Although statisticians are working on methods to do this [83, 90, 109], we still lack a method that addresses the complexity inherent in multiple QOL component data. It is important to remember that it may not be as informative to combine components as to examine them separately. Individual QOL components identify the exact type of functioning deficit or improvement that occurred.

Finally, one other method of weighting or adjusting patient QOL data is the QALYs technique. Researchers [56, 111] have developed methods for weighting years gained in survival by one treatment versus another with respect to the quality of those years. This approach requires information on patient preferences for different health states (obtained through a variety of methods such as the standard gamble). Such data form the basis for utility functions used to weight life years. This approach has yet to be used specifically with pain reports but, given access to preference or valuations of pain/health states, it may prove useful. Obtaining patient valuation of reported health/QOL states is a complicated, usually resource-intensive process.

Conclusions

Research on cancer pain and its relief is far more difficult than study of postoperative or other severe pain. Cancer-related pain arises from many causes and degrades all aspects of life for weeks, months or even years. Controlling the pain associated with cancer and its treatment means more than symptom management for it determines whether life is precious or an unbearable burden. Therapeutic outcome research directed at improving the control of cancer pain addresses more than the patient's reported pain relief. Successful pain control protects and sustains the quality of the patient's life.

Traditionally, such concerns have fallen outside the scope of cancer pain research. Researchers have lacked the necessary tools for assessing patients comprehensively and across large windows of time. Our review indicates that QOL researchers have developed assessment tools that can permit comprehensive, multidimensional evaluation of patient well-being over time as a function of pain control.

Despite the momentum and strong progress in QOL research overall, this frontier will not yield easily to pioneer pain researchers who elect to explore it. Causal attribution issues in constantly changing and complex circumstances, measurement difficulties, and design quandaries present formidable challenges to the evaluation of pain management strategies. Moreover, there are undoubtedly many QOL problems specific to pain research that we have failed to foresee. And because this approach to clinical research departs from tradition, communication barriers may limit the impact of progress in pain related QOL research.

Despite these problems, we conclude that a QOL approach to therapeutic outcome questions in the cancer pain field is both timely and feasible. As long as an investigator specifies in advance a reasonable number of QOL components as the basis for treatment arm comparisons (and that will almost always include traditional pain assessment endpoints), the study of QOL will shed light on the multidimensional value of a pain-relieving intervention. It is likely that multidimensional evaluation will become the rule rather than the exception in cancer pain research, in part because of the precedents set by QOL studies.

Perhaps the principal value of QOL research for the pain field is its multidimensional nature. QOL research strategies may compel clinical pain control investigators to conceptualize research questions more broadly and comprehensively. QOL researchers, in the spirit of Edwin Abbott [7] are likely to "...stir up a race of rebels who shall refuse to be confined to limited dimensionality."

References

1. Aaronson NK, Bullinger M, Ahmedzai S (1988) A modular approach to quality-of-life assessment in cancer clinical trials. Recent Results Cancer Res 111: 231–249
2. Aaronson NK (1988) Quality of life: what is it? How should it be measured? Oncology 2: 69–74
3. Aaronson NK (1990) Quality of life research in cancer clinical trials: a need for common rules and language. Oncology 4: 59–66
4. Aaronson NK, Bakker W, Stewart AL et al (1987) Multidimensional approach to the measurement of quality of life in lung cancer clinical trials. In: Aaronson NK, Beckmann JH (eds) Monograph series of the European Organization for Research and Treatment of Cancer, vol. 17. Raven Press, New York, pp 63–82
5. Aaronson N, Calais da Silva F, Denis L, et al (1989) Quality of life in patients with muscle-infiltrating bladder cancer and hormone-resistant prostatic cancer. Eur Urol 16: 335–339

6. Allen MG, Yen WM (1979) Introduction to measurement theory. Brooks/Cole Publ Co, Monterey, CA
7. Abbott EA (1963) Flatland: A romance of many dimensions. New York, Barnes & Noble, p. 7
8. Andrews FM, Withey SB (eds) (1976) Social indicators of well-being. Plenum Press, New York
9. Barofsky I, Sugarbaker PH (1990) Cancer. In: Spilker B (ed) Quality of life assessment in clinical trials. Raven Press, New York, pp 419–439
10. Bearman SK, Appelbaum FR, Buckner CD, et al (1988) Regimen-related toxicity in patients undergoing bone marrow transplantation. J Clin Oncol 6: 1562–1568
11. Beyer JE, Wells N (1989) The assessment of pain in children. Ped Clin N Am 36: 837–854
12. Bonica JJ (ed) (1990) The management of pain, 2nd edition. Lea & Febiger, Philadelphia
13. Brody DS (1980) Physician recognition of behavioral, psychosocial, and social aspects of medical care. Arch Intern Med 140: 1286–1289
14. Brown CH (1990) Protecting against nonrandomly missing data in longitudinal studies. Biometrics 46: 143–155
15. Campbell A, Converse PE, Rodgers WL (eds) (1976) The quality of American life. Sage, New York
16. Campbell DT, Fiske DW (1959) Convergent and discriminant validation by the multitrait-multimethod matrix. Psychol Bull 56: 81–105
17. Cassell EJ (1982) The nature of suffering and the goals of medicine. N Engl J Med 306: 639–645
18. Cassell EJ (ed) (1985) The healer's art. MIT Press, Cambridge MA
19. Cella DF, Cherin EA (1987) Measuring quality of life in patients with cancer. In: Proceedings of the fifth national conference on human values and cancer. New York, Am Cancer Soc, pp 23–31
20. Cella DF, Tulsky DS (1990) Measuring quality of life today: methodological aspects. Oncology 4: 29–38
21. Chambers LW, MacDonald LA, Tugwell R, et al (1982) The McMaster Health Index Questionnaire as a measure of quality of life for patients with rheumatoid disease. J Rheumatol 7: 780–784
22. Chapman CR, Syrjala KS, Sargur M (1985) Pain as a manifestation of cancer treatment. Sem Nurs Oncol 1: 100–108
23. Chapman CR, Syrjala KL (1990) Measurement of pain. In: Bonica JJ (ed) The management of pain, 2nd ed. Lea & Febiger, Philadelphia, pp 580–594
24. Clark A, Fallowfield LJ (1986) Quality of life measurements in patients with malignant disease. J R Soc Med 79: 165–169
25. Clarridge BR, Massagli MP (1989) The use of female spouse proxies in common symptom reporting. Med Care 27: 352–366
26. Cleeland CS (1985) Measurement and prevalence of pain in cancer. Semin Oncol Nurs 1: 87–92
27. Coyle N, Foley K (1987) Prevalence and profile of pain syndromes in cancer patients. In: McGuire DB, Yarbro CH (eds) Cancer pain management. Grune and Stratton, New York, pp 21–46
28. Cronbach LJ (1951) Coefficient alpha and the internal structure of tests. Psymtrka 16: 297–334
29. Daut RL, Cleeland CS, Flanery RC (1983) Development of the Wisconsin Brief Pain Questionnaire to assess pain in cancer and other diseases. Pain 17: 197–210
30. de Haes JCJM, van Knippenberg FCE (1987) Quality of life of cancer patients. Review of the literature. In: Aaronson NK, Beckmann JH (eds) The quality of life of cancer patients. Raven Press, New York, pp 167–182
31. de Haes JCJM, van Oostrom MA, Welvaart K (1986) The effect of radical and conserving surgery on the quality of life of early breast cancer patients. Eur J Surg Oncol 12: 337–342

32. de Haes JCJM, Raatgever JW, van der Burg MEL, et al (1987) Evaluation of the quality of life of patients with advanced ovarian cancer treated with combination chemotherapy. In: Aaronson NK, Beckmann JH (eds) Monograph series of the European Organization for Research and Treatment of Cancer, vol 17. Raven Press, New York, pp 215–226
33. de Haes JC, van Knippenberg FC (1989) Quality of life instruments for cancer patients: "Babel's Tower" revisited. J Clin Epidemiol 42: 1239–41
34. Derogatis L, Melisaratos N (1983) The Brief Symptom Inventory: an introductory report. Psychol Med 13: 1–10
35. Derogatis LR (1986) The Psychosocial Adjustment to Illness Scale (PAIS). J Psychosom Res 30: 77–91
36. Deyo RA, Diehr P, Patrick DL Reproducibility and responsiveness of health status measures: statistics and strategies for evaluation. Controlled Clin Trials (in press)
37. Donovan K, Sanson-Fisher RW, Redman S (1989) Measuring quality of life in cancer patients. J Clin Oncol 7: 959–968
38. Elliott K, Foley KM (1990) Neurologic pain syndromes in patients with cancer. Crit Care Clin 6: 393–420
39. Fayers PM, Jones DR (1983) Measuring and analyzing quality of life in cancer clinical trials: a review. Stat med 2: 429–446
40. Ferrans CE (1990) Development of a quality of life index for patients with cancer. Oncol Nurs Forum 17: 15–19
41. Ferrans CE, Power MJ (1985) Quality of life index: development and psychometric properties. Adv Nurs Sci 8: 15–24
42. Fishman B, Pasternak S, Wallenstein SL, et al (1987) The Memorial Pain Assessment Card: a valid instrument for evaluation of cancer pain (abstr). Cancer 60: 1151–1158
43. Frank-Stromberg M (1984) Selecting an instrument to measure quality of life. Oncol Nurs Forum 11: 88–91
44. Ganz PA, Rofessart J, Polinsky ML, et al (1986) A comprehensive approach to the assessment of cancer patients' rehabilitation needs: the Cancer Inventory of Problem Situations and a companion interview. J Psychosoc Oncol 4: 27–42
45. Geddes DM, Dones L, Hill E, et al (1990) Quality of life during chemotherapy for small cell lung cancer: assessment and use of a daily diary card in a randomized trial. Eur J Cancer 26: 484–492
46. Goldhirsh A, Gelber RD, Simes RJ, et al (1989) Costs and benefits of adjuvant therapy in breast cancer: a quality-adjusted survival analysis. J Clin Oncol 7: 36–44
47. Guyatt G, Walter S, Norman G (1987) Measuring change over time: assessing the usefulness of evaluative instruments. J Chronic Dis 40: 171–178
48. Guyatt GH, Deyo RA, Charlson M, et al (1989) Responsiveness and validity in health status measurement: a clarification. J Clin Epidemiol 42: 403–408
49. Harkins SW, Kwentus J, Price DD (1990) Pain and suffering in the elderly. In: Bonica JJ (ed) The management of pain, 2nd ed. Lea & Febiger, Philadelphia, pp 552–559
50. Heinrich RL, Schag CC, Ganz PA (1984) Living with cancer: the Cancer Inventory of Problem Situations. J Clin Psychol 40: 972–980
51. Hollandsworth JG Jr (1988) Evaluating the impact of medical treatment on quality of life: a 5-year update. Soc Sci Med 26: 425–434
52. Hunt SM, McKenna SP, McEwen J, et al (1981) The Nottingham Health Profiles: subjective health status and medical consultations. Soc Sci Med 15: 221–229
53. International Association for the Study of Pain (1986) Pain terms: a current list with definitions and notes on usage. Pain 3 [Suppl]: S 216
54. Jeans ME (1983) The measurement of pain in children. In: R Melzack (ed) Pain measurement and assessment. Raven Press, New York, p 183–189
55. Kaplan RS, Wiernik PH (1982) Neurotoxicity of antineoplastic drugs. Semin Oncol 9: 103–130
56. Kaplan RM, Anderson JP (1988) A Central Health Policy Model: update and applications. HSR: Health Serv Res 23: 203–235

57. Kaplan RM, Anderson JP (1990) The Central Health Policy Model: an integrated approach. In: Spilker B (ed) Quality of life assessments in clinical trials. Raven Press, New York, pp 131149
58. Karnofsky DA, Burchenal JH (1949) The clinical evaluation of chemotherapeutic agents in cancer. In: MacLeod CM (ed) Evaluation of chemotherapeutic agents. Columbia Univ Press, New York, pp 191–205
59. Kori S, Foley KM, Posner JB (1981) Brachial plexus lesions in patients with cancer: 100 cases. Neurology 35: 3–15
60. Lee VC, Rowlingson JC (1990) Chronic pain management. In: Spilker B (ed) Quality of life assessments in clinical trials. Raven Press, New York, pp 269–293
61. Levine MN, Guyatt GH, Gent M, et al (1988) Quality of life in stage II breast cancer: an instrument for clinical trials. J Clin Oncol 6: 1798–1810
62. Liang MH, Katz JN, Ginsburg KS (1990) Chronic rheumatic disease. In: Spilker B (ed) Quality of life assessments in clinical trials. Raven Press, New York, pp 441–458
63. Magaziner J, Simonsick EM, Kashner TM et al. (1988) Patient-proxy response comparability on measures of patient health and functional status. J Clin Epidemiol 41: 1065–1074
64. Martin DP, Gilson BS, Bergner M, et al (1976) The Sickness Impact Profile: potential use of a health status instrument for physician training. J Med Educ 51: 942–944
65. Martini CJ, McDowell I (1976) Health status: patient and physician judgments. Health Serv Res 11: 508–515
66. McCorkle R, Young K (1978) Development of a symptom distress scale. Cancer Nurs 1: 373–378
67. McCorkle R, Benoliel JQ (1983) Symptom distress, current concerns and mood disturbance after diagnosis of life-threatening disease. Soc Sci Med 17: 431–438
68. McCorkle R (1987) The measurement of symptom distress. Semin Oncol Nurs 3: 248–256
69. McCorkle R, Benoliel JQ, Donaldson G, et al (1989) A randomized clinical trial of home nursing care for lung cancer patients. Cancer 64: 1375–1382
70. McGrath PA (1990) Pain assessment in children – A practical approach. In: Tyler DC, Krane EJ (eds) Advances in pain research and therapy, vol 15. Raven Press, New York, pp 5–30
71. McGrath PA, Mathews JR, Pigeon BA (Submitted) Assessment of pain in children: a systematic psychosocial model.
72. Meenan RF (1982) The AIMS approach to health status measurement: conceptual background and measurement properties. J Rheumatol 9: 785–788
73. Melzack R (1975) The McGill Pain Questionnaire: major properties and scoring methods. Pain 1: 277–299
74. Melzack R (1981) The shortform McGill Pain Questionaire. Pain 30: 191–197
75. Moinpour CM, Feigl P, Metch B, et al (1989) Quality of life end points in cancer clinical trials: review and recommendations. J Natl Cancer Inst 81: 485–495
76. Moinpour CM, Donaldson G, Wallace K, et al (1990) Parent/child agreement in rating child mouth pain. In: Tyler DC, Krane EJ (eds) Advances in pain research and therapy, vol 15. Raven Press, New York, pp 69–78
77. Moinpour CM, Hayden KA, Thompson IM (1990) Quality of life assessment in southwest oncology group trials. Oncology 4: 79–89
78. Monks R, Taenzer P (1983) A comprehensive pain questionnaire. In: Melzack R (ed) Pain measurement and assessment. Raven Press, New York, pp 233–237, 1A–14A
79. Najman JM, Levine S (1981) Evaluating the impact of medical care and technologies on the quality of life: a review and critique. Soc Sci Med 15: 107–115
80. National Cancer Institute (1990) Recommendations of working group on assessment issues, quality of life in cancer clinical trials, July 16–17, Unpublished Conference Report
81. Nelson E, Conger B, Douglass R, et al (1983) Functional health status levels of primary care patients. JAMA 249: 3331–3338
82. Nunnally JC (ed) (1978) Psychometric Theory. McGraw Hill Book Co, New York

83. Olschewski M, Schumacher M (1990) Statistical analysis of quality of life data in cancer clinical trials. Stat Med 9: 749–763
84. Padilla GV, Ferrell B, Grant MM, et al (1990) Defining the content domain of quality of life for cancer patients with pain. Cancer Nurs 13: 108–115
85. Palmer JJ (1972) Radiation myelopathy. Brain 95: 109–122
86. Patrick DL, Deyo RA (1989) Generic and disease-specific measures in assessing health status and quality of life. Med Care 27: S217–S232
87. Patrick DL, Erickson P (1988) What constitutes quality of life? Concepts and dimensions. Clin Nutr 7: 53–63
88. Patterson KL, Klopovich PM (1987) Pain in the pediatric oncology patient. In: McGuire DB, Yarbro CH (eds) Cancer pain management. Grune & Stratton, Orlando, p 259–272
89. Payne R (1990) Pathophysiology of cancer pain. In: Foley KM, Bonica JJ, Ventafridda V (eds) Advances in pain research and therapy (proceedings of the second international congress on cancer pain), vol 16. Raven Press, New York, pp 13–26
90. Pocock SJ, Geller NL, Tsiatis AA (1987) The analysis of multiple endpoints in clinical trials. Biometrics 43: 487–498
91. Portenoy RK (1990) Pain and quality of life: Clinical issues and implications for research. Oncology 4: 172–178
92. Press OW, Schaller RT Jr (1987) Thomas ED, Bone marrow transplant complications. In: Toledo-Pereyra LH (ed) Complications of organ transplantation. Marcel Dekker, New York, pp 399–424
93. Ross DM, Ross SA (1988) Childhood pain. Current issues, research, and management. Urban & Schwarzenberg, Baltimore, pp 111–166
94. Rotstein J, Good RA (1957) Steroid pseudorheumatism. Arch Intern Med 99: 545–555
95. Rubin P (1983) Statement of the clinical oncologic problem. In: Rubin P (ed) Clinical oncology: A multidisciplinary approach, 6th ed. Rochester, NY, American Cancer Society, pp 2–19
96. Schag CC, Heinrich RL (1990) Development of a comprehensive quality of life measurement tool: CARES. Oncology 4: 135–138
97. Schag CC, Heinrich RL, Aadland RL, et al (1990) Assessing problems of cancer patients: psychometric properties of the Cancer Inventory of Problem Situations. Health Psychol 9: 83–102
98. Schipper H (1990) Guidelines and caveats for quality of life measurement in clinical practice and research. Oncology 4: 51–57
99. Selby P, Robertson B (1987) Measurement of quality of life in patients with cancer. Cancer Surv 6: 521–543
100. Shimamura Y, Gunven P, Takenaka Y, et al (1988) Combined peripheral and central chemoembolization of liver tumors. Experience with Lipiodol-Doxorubicin and gelatin sponge (L-TAE). Cancer 61: 238–242
101. Shumaker SA, Anderson RT, Czajkowski SM (1990) Psychological tests and scales. In: Spilker B (ed) Quality of life assessment in clinical trials. Raven Press, New York, pp 95–113
102. Slevin ML, Plant H, Lynch D, et al (1988) Who should measure quality of life, the doctor or the patient? Br J Cancer 57: 109–112
103. Sonis A, Sonis S (1979) Oral complications of cancer chemotherapy in pediatric patients. J Periodon 3: 122–128
104. Spitzer WO, Dobson AJ, Hall J, et al (1981) Measuring the quality of life of cancer patients. A concise QL-Index for use by physicians. J Chronic Dis 34: 585–597
105. Stewart AL, Hays RD, Ware JE Jr (1988) The MDS Short-form General Health Survey. Reliability and validity in a patient population. Med Care 26: 724–735
106. Stewart AL, Greenfield S, Hays RD, et al (1989) Functional status and well-being of patients with chronic conditions. Results from The Medical Outcomes Study. JAMA 262: 907–913

107. Stjernsward J, Teoh N (1990) The scope of the cancer pain problem. In: Foley KM, Bonica JJ, Ventafridda V (eds) Advances in pain research and therapy (proceedings of the second international congress on cancer pain), vol 16. Raven Press, New York, pp 7–12
108. Strang P, Qvarner H (1990) Cancer-related pain and its influence on quality of life. Anticancer Res 10: 109–112
109. Tandon PK (1990) Applications of global statistics in analysing quality of life data. Stat Med 9: 819–827
110. Tannock I, Gospdoarowica M, Meakin W, et al (1989) Treatment of metastatic prostatic cancer with low-dose prednisone: evaluation of pain and quality of life as pragmatic indices of response. J Clin Oncol 7: 590–597
111. Torrance GW, Feeny D (1989) Utilities and quality-adjusted life years. Intl J Technol Assess Hlth Care 5: 559–575
112. Twycross RG, Fairfield S (1982) Pain in far advanced cancer. Pain 14: 303–310
113. Twycross RG, Lack SA (1983) Symptom control in far advanced cancer: Pain Relief. Pitman Books Ltd, London
114. Tyler DC (1990) Pain in infants and children. In: Bonica JJ (ed) The management of pain, 2nd ed. Lea & Febiger, Philadelphia, pp 538–551
115. Ware JE Jr (1987) Standards for validating health measures: definition and content. J Chronic Dis 40: 473–480
116. Ware JE Jr (1990) Health related domains of quality of life. Paper presented at Quality of Life Research in Cancer Clinical Trials, National Cancer Institute Workshop, July 16–17
117. Wartman SA, Morlock LL, Malitz FE, et al (1983) Impact of divergent evaluations by physicians and patients of patient's complaints. Public Health Rep 98: 141–145
118. Willis WD (ed) (1985) Pain and headache [The pain system: The neuro basis of nociceptive transmission in the mammalian nervous system], vol 8. Karger, New York
119. World Health Organization (1958) The first ten years of the World Health Organization. Geneva, WHO
120. World Health Organization (1979) WHO handbook for reporting results of cancer treatment. Offset Publ No 48, WHO, Geneva
121. World Health Organization (1980) International classification of impairments, disabilities and handicaps. WHO, Geneva
122. Young KJ, Longman AJ (1983) Quality of life and persons with melanoma: a pilot study. Cancer Nurs 6: 219–225
123. Zubrod CG, Schneiderman M, Frei E, et al (1960) Appraisal methods for the study of chemotherapy of cancer in man: comparative therapeutic trial of nitrogen mustard and triethylene thiophosphoramide. J Chronic Dis 11: 7–33

Opioid Analgesia for Chronic, Nonmalignant Pain

M. Strumpf and M. Zenz

Introduction

Reports in the literature on the use of opioids in chronic pain not attributable to cancer are few [1, 5, 6, 10, 11, 12, 14, 15]. In 1986 Portenoy and Foley [6] reported on the use of opioids in nonmalignant pain, and the World Congresses of the IASP devoted a session to this subject in 1987 and 1990. The indication for opioids in patients suffering from extreme, incurable pain has been the theme of controversial discussions [1, 4]. Long-term therapy with opioids is surrounded by prejudice with regard to sedation, addiction, or the inevitable development of tolerance.

Methods

During the period from May 1986 to May 1990, we gave opioid therapy to a total of 100 patients suffering from extreme, nonmalignant pain. These patients suffered from:

- Neuropathic pain ($n = 53$)
- Back pain ($n = 24$)
- Osteoporosis ($n = 11$)
- Head and facial pain ($n = 8$)
- Ischemic pain ($n = 2$)
- Rheumatic pain ($n = 2$).

Only when all possible alternative treatments had failed to achieve effective pain reduction were opiods used (e.g., exhaustion of all therapeutic possibilities with regard to cause, failure of specific therapy in specific types of pain, exclusion of psychogenesis of the pain, settling of surgical or neurosurgical procedures, and the use of non-narcotic drugs including psychoactive drugs).

In patients who had never before been treated with opioids, we began with weak opioids, usually with sustained-release dihydrocodeine (DHC Continus, Napp) at an initial dose of 2×60 mg daily.

If weak opioids had already been used and tolerated, without producing any clear pain-reducing effect, we started by giving buprenorphine at an initial dose of 3 × 1 tablet (3 × 0.2 mg) sublingually. The dose was increased as required to achieve pain reduction. If a daily dose of more than 4 × 6 tablets of buprenorphine was needed we changed to sustained-release morphine tablets at an initial dose of 3 × 30 mg. If pain reduction was still inadequate, we doubled the dose of sustained-release morphine (e.g., 3 × 60 mg) in intervals of 3–4 days, until the patients achieved effective pain reduction or side effects became predominant.

Visual analogue scales (VAS) were used in assessing pain reduction [8]. For each individual patient two different values of VAS were used: (a) the sum of eight VAS values (every 2 h from 8 a.m. to 10 p.m.) of every day (SVAS) and (b) the peak value of the VAS of every day (PVAS). Efficacy of treatment was registered by allocation to the following three categories: good relief (≥ 50 % pain reduction), partial pain relief (between 25 % and 50 % pain reduction), and nonresponders (<25 % pain reduction). Treatment effects were recorded on days 1, 3, 5, 7, 14, and 21 after commencement of opioid therapy. Success of the treatment was subsequently monitored at greater intervals (every month).

Karnofsky's "general performance status" [3] was used to determine the patient's performance.

Adverse reactions were recorded at regular intervals. Criteria for discontinuation were inefficacy of opiate therapy, therapy-resistant adverse reactions, lack of compliance, and death.

Results

The patients investigated included 53 men and 47 women with an average age of 59.1 years (range 29–81 years). The mean duration of treatment was 224 days (range 14–1 472 days). The total duration of treatment for all patients was 22 421 days, equivalent to 61.4 patient years.

Thirteen patients had already been treated for pain for over 20 years, 33 patients for 10 to 20 years, 31 patients for 5 to 10 years, 22 patients for 1 to 5 years and only one patient for less than 1 year.

Drugs had been prescribed for all 100 patients before the study began. Non-narcotic analgesics, compound analgesic preparations (in most cases), opioids and/or psychotropic drugs had been given. Previous treatments with strong or weak opioids had not, with one exception, been performed according to a time schedule, but "as required" to control pain. A total of 358 weeks of hospitalization had been required during previous treatment.

In our study, 57 patients were given buprenorphine. Of 23 patients who we treated with sustained-release morphine, 13 had previously been taking buprenorphine (inadequate pain reduction). Nineteen patients were given sustained-release dihydrocodeine, 1 patient methadone (Fig. 1).

The further results relate only to the SVAS values because of a close correlation between SVAS and PVAS values: In 51 patients, a reduction of pain ≥ 50 % was achieved after 14 days of therapy. Twenty-eight patients

	Dihydrocodeine SR	Buprenorphine	Morphine SR
n	19	57	23
x (mg)	170	1.46	255
Range (mg)	60–540	0.4–3.2	20–2 000

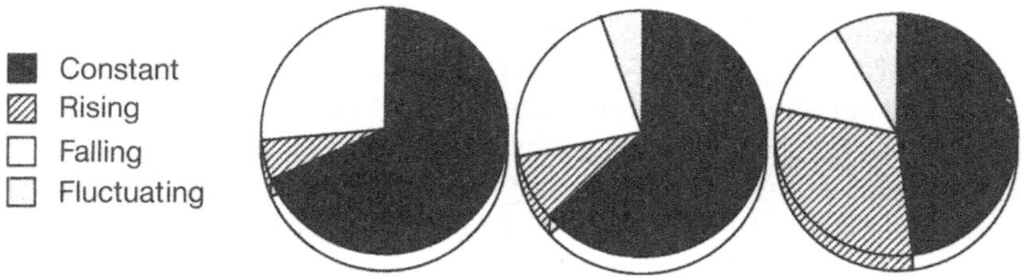

Fig. 1. Comparison of dosages of opioids used

responded to opioids with a 25 %–50 % pain reduction, which was described subjectively as definite relief. In 21 cases, opioids were found to be ineffective [Fig. 2].

Performance for the whole population improved with opioid therapy, particularly in the 51 patients who reacted to opioids with at least 50 % pain reduction. This subgroup improved from a mean Karnofsky index of 65 (1 %) to 79 (4 %). In the nonresponder group the Karnofsky index fell from a mean of 71 (3 %) to 61 (9 %). There was a positive correlation ($p < 0.001$) between the pain reduction (SVAS) and the increase of the performance.

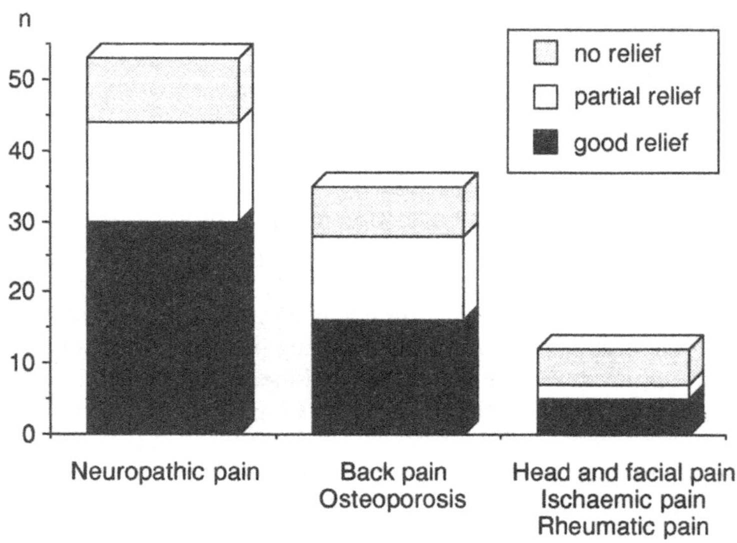

Fig. 2. Diagnoses and pain reduction (N = 100/SVAS) 14 days after start of therapy

Constipation, fatigue, dizziness, nausea with occasional vomiting, itching, and micturition difficulties were recorded. At the start of therapy, 38 patients complained of constipation, 28 of fatigue, 41 of dizziness, 30 of nausea and five of itching or micturition difficulties. At the end of the observation period, 46 patients reported constipation. All other adverse reactions decreased markedly. In those patients with good pain relief, overall adverse reactions were less marked. Respiratory depression and euphoria were not seen in any patient, even in the nonresponder category.

Discussion

Indication

The following common features emerged from our patients' case histories: (a) long treatment periods, (b) a high proportion of time spent in hospital, (c) the large number of doctors who had previously given treatment, (d) polypragmasy of therapy including recourse to massive destructive neurosurgical procedures, (e) the misuse of unsuitable drugs which produced dependence, sedation or agitation in the patients without achieving pain reduction, (f) the use of weak opioids at irregular intervals "as required to control the pain", (g) the withholding of effective drugs for fear of developing addiction, and (h) tolerance, sedation or respiratory depression.

Opioids in many cases provide satisfactory analgesia for patients who have undergone years of unsuccessful therapy. In accordance with the findings of our studies on tumor pain [16, 17], patients with nonmalignant pain can also safely be given long-term treatment with opioids.

Our data indicate that opioids may also be effective in neuropathic pain. In more than half of our patients suffering in this way we observed good pain reduction. In contrast to this result, we found that the patients with head and facial pain achieved significantly ($p < 0.01$) less pain relief than the group with neuropathic pain (Fig. 3).

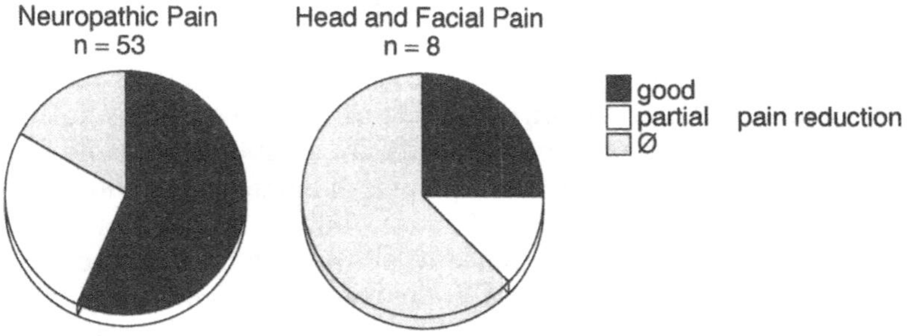

Fig. 3. Pain reduction (SVAS) 14 days after start of therapy (neuropathic pain vs head and facial pain)

Performance

In the pharmacological literature, sedation and anguish are described as adverse reactions to opiate therapy [2]. By contrast, other authors [13] report improved performance and activity and decreasing passivity of tumor patients taking opioids for pain. This is also true, as shown by the present study, for opioid therapy in nonmalignant pain: the performance was best in patients with good pain reduction; it fell only in the group of nonresponders.

Side effects

Almost all opioids produce adverse reactions, but these are generally manageable and nonhazardous. Prevention of constipation is obligatory, since this becomes an increasing problem during the course of opiate therapy [13]. An appropriate diet, together with oral and rectal laxatives, are indicated. A combination of other adverse reactions such as fatigue, nausea, vomiting and dizziness may occur in the initial phase, but generally subside in the course of treatment.

Psychological and Physical Dependence

In most of the studies we find the term "addiction" to describe physical dependence as well as psychological dependence. In the literature, addiction rates from 0.03 % [7] to 17 % [11] are reported. Addiction to opioids is widely assumed, but is not documented for carefully treated patients. Our own experiences demonstrate that psychological dependence is an extraordinarily rare occurrence [16, 17]. In our investigation none of the 59 patients in whom therapy was stopped had psychological symptoms of drug-seeking behavior after opioid therapy. The basis for this result is a systematic therapy according to a time schedule [13], which must, of course, also be applied in patients with nonmalignant, incurable pain. The pain periods of a chronic pain patient treated with opioids "as required" are similar to the period of dysphoria of a street addict. Both groups have recurrent pain or discomfort because of too long intervals between drug administration, as well as a craving for the next drug application (addiction).

Physical dependence is characterized by tolerance effects and by withdrawal symptoms after abruption of opioid therapy. Opioids show tolerance which is "selective" [10]: they produce analgesia, fatigue, nausea and constipation. Fatigue and nausea subside in the course of opiate treatment, after about 2–3 weeks. This does indicate tolerance, but it should not necessarily be concluded that general tolerance to all the effects of opiates will develop. Constipation tends to increase in the course of opioid therapy. There is no tolerance in this respect. On dose reduction, no withdrawal symptoms were seen in our population. After withdrawal of therapy only mild (physical) withdrawal symptoms were registered.

Narcotics legislation

In the Federal Republic of Germany, opioids are subject to unreasonable restrictions and provisos with regard to prescription. Doctors are deterred from applying for and making out prescriptions for narcotics, not only by controversy over the risk of addiction in pain patients but also by the administrative cost arising from legislative requirements and fear of prescription thefts. Only 16 % of general practitioners prescribe strong opioid analgesics, even when there is a basic indication for opioids [9]. These strict narcotics regulations in the medical sphere have not, however, had the desired effect on the availability of illegal drugs; the rising number of deaths from drugs of first-time users and drug delinquents leads to the conclusion that the drugs scene cannot be influenced by narcotics legislation. The necessary therapeutic care of many patients suffering from pain is clearly hindered by these regulations.

Alternative to Opioid Therapy

Most of the patients we investigated had previously received psychoactive drugs for pain control. In spite of the serious adverse reactions, such drugs are widely prescribed without hesitation for patients with extreme pain. The altered impression of pain associated with an improvement in the subjective feeling of well-being must not be misinterpreted as an analgesic effect. Nor does the additional use of psychoactive drugs allow a reduction in opioids or potentiation of the opioid effect. Antidepressants and neuroleptics are indicated only in neuropathic pain syndromes with a predominantly dysesthetic pain component. Psychoactive drugs should therefore be used in pain therapy only where they are strictly indicated.

Conclusion

Indication of opioid therapy is determined by the severity of the pain and not by diagnosis. This must also be true for pain in an underlying disease which is nonmalignant. Incurable pain is not only found in cancer patients. A refractory, extreme pain – even when occurring in a benign underlying disorder – must in many cases be assessed as "malignant" on the basis of quality and intensity.

The rules for opioid administration with which we are familiar in the treatment of cancer pain must also be adhered to in patients with nonmalignant pain. The first of these is administration according to a time schedule and not "as required". The patient must be monitored continuously.

Psychogenesis of pain must be excluded before opioid therapy is selected. Causal therapy, of course, always takes precedence over the possible use of opioids. However, there is no justification for withholding opioids from patients when all other therapeutic measures have failed.

References

1. Arnér A, Meyerson B (1988) Lack of analgesic effect of opioids on neuropathic and idiopathic forms of pain. Pain 33: 11–24
2. Jaffe JH (1986) Drug addiction and drug abuse. In: Goodman Gilman A, Goodman LS, Rall TW, Murad F (eds). The pharmacological basis of therapeutics. Macmillan, New York Toronto London, p 532
3. Karnofsky DA, Abelman WH, Craver LF, Burchenal JH (1948) The use of the nitrogen mustards in the palliative treatment of carcinoma. Cancer 1: 634–656
4. Keup W (1988) Chronische Einnahme von Opioid-Analgetika bei Schmerzsyndromen nicht-maligner Ursache. Bericht über 38 Fälle. Kommentar zur Arbeit von Portenoy und Foley. Schmerz 2: 167–169
5. Portenoy RK (1990) Chronic opioid therapy in nonmalignant pain. J Pain Sympt Management 5 (suppl 1): 46–62
6. Portenoy PK, Foley KM (1986) Chronic use of opioid analgesics in non-malignant pain: report of 38 cases. Pain 25: 171–186
7. Porter JH, Jick J (1980) Addiction rare in patients treated with narcotics. New Engl J Med 302: 123
8. Scott DB, Huskisson EC (1976) Graphic representation of pain. Pain 2: 175
9. Sorge J, Zenz M (1989) Schmerzpatienten unterversorgt. Verschreibung von Betäubungsmitteln: Vorurteile und Hindernisse. Ein Vergleich 1985–1988. Dt Ärzteblatt 86: A 2231–2234
10. Taub A (1982) Opioid analgesics in the treatment of chronic intractable pain of non-neoplastic origin. In: Kitahata LM, Collins D (eds). Narcotic analgesics in anaesthesiology. Williams and Wilkens, Baltimore; pp 199–208
11. Tennant FS, Robinson D, Sagherian A, Seecof R (1988) Chronic opioid treatment on intractable, non-malignant pain. NIDA Res Monogr 81: 174–180
12. Tennant FS, Uelmen GF (1983) Narcotic maintenance for chronic pain: medical and legal guidelines. Postgraduate medicine J 73: 81–94
13. Twycross RG (1988) Opioid analgesics in cancer pain: current practice and controversies. Cancer Surveys 7: 29–53
14. Urban BJ, France RD, Steinberger DL, Scott DL, Maltbie AA (1986) Long-term use of narcotic/antidepressant medication in the management of phantom limb pain. Pain 24: 191–197
15. Wan Lu C, Urban B, France RD (1988) Long-term narcotic therapy in chronic pain. Presented at the Canadian Pain Society and American Pain Society, Joint Meeting, Toronto, Canada, November 10–13
16. Zenz M, Piepenbrock S, Tryba M, Glocke M, Everlin M, Klauke W (1985) Langzeittherapie von Krebsschmerzen – Kontrollierte Studie mit Buprenorphin. Dtsch med Wschr 110: 448–453
17. Zenz M, Strumpf M, Tryba M, Steffmann B, Röhrs E (1989) Retardiertes Morphin zur Langzeittherapie schwerer Tumorschmerzen. Dtsch med. Wschr 114: 43–47

Part III. Noninvasive Fentanyl Application

Pharmacokinetics of Fentanyl

L. E. MATHER and G. K. GOURLAY

Introduction

The fundamental pharmacokinetic properties of any drug are the rate and extent of distribution in the body and the rate and route(s) of elimination from the body. These, as a rule, are determined after intravenous administration. As reported in a variety of studies using traditional compartment pharmacokinetic methodology over the past 10 years, the fundamental pharmacokinetic properties of fentanyl in adult humans are not complex. On average, these properties consist of an extensive extravascular distribution (total apparent volume of distribution, Vss = 300–400 l/70 kg), a medium to high total body clearance (0.5–1.2 l/min), and a low renal clearance (urinary excretion <10% dose), and are consistent with the lipophilic tertiary amine chemical structure of fentanyl. It is noteworthy that there is a large variability in the results of different investigations and there may be many reasons for this. Assay differences may account for some of the problems. At the doses used, blood fentanyl concentrations after intravenous bolus are not readily measurable with accuracy by specific chemical methods over a sufficient range, and immunoassay methods still leave residual concerns about specificity. Undoubtedly, some of the variability in reported pharmacokinetics of fentanyl also derives from differences in the samples assayed (e.g., arterial or venous blood, plasma or serum; and drug sorption), differences in the physiological status of the subjects (e.g., age, pathology, binding proteins, concomitant drugs, anesthesia and surgery) and differences in the mode of fentanyl administration (e.g., bolus, infusion). With some exceptions, these variables have not been examined systematically, but it is clear from first principles that each could be significant.

Because of a short duration of action of single doses, fentanyl was originally thought to have a short plasma half-life due to rapid metabolism. It has since been shown that the "short plasma half-life" was due to drug assays insufficiently sensitive to follow drug concentrations for long enough to determine the true value, and it was due more to extravascular distribution than clearance, anyway. In fact, the average plasma half-life (6–10 h) derives

The support of the National Health and Medical Research Council of Australia is acknowledged not from the rate of metabolism but from washout of poorly perfused tissues (principally fat) which have a high capacity for fentanyl uptake. Fentanyl has been shown to undergo extensive pulmonary uptake (approximately 80%) during first pass through the lungs. This is not uncommon among lipophilic amines and, presumably, is due to the range of pulmonary transit times, reversible binding, and ion-trapping in lung water; it serves to spread and attenuate the arrival of drug concentrations in arterial blood. The "sequestered" drug is released rapidly (in minutes) and there is no convincing evidence that fentanyl is metabolized in lung tissue in vivo.

If the drug is introduced into the body by some process involving absorption, then the rate and extent of the absorption process(es) become of interest also. Intramuscular injection of fentanyl would not have any clinical advantage and would be expected to produce as unpredictable a response as that shown for IM pethidine. As the liver is the putative principal region of fentanyl clearance, oral fentanyl has poor bioavailability due to high hepatosplanchnic clearance. Secondary blood concentration peaks, which have been suggested as being due to absorption of gastric juice "ion-trapped" fentanyl, are more likely to occur because of fentanyl washout from nonvisceral tissues than because of fentanyl's gastric recycling. Recently, use has been made of the high lipid solubility of fentanyl base in the development of oral-buccal- and sublingual dosage forms. Inhalation of nebulized fentanyl produces sustained blood drug concentrations consistent with about 10% bioavailability. In each case, it would be expected that swallowed fentanyl would contribute little to the blood drug concentrations, making each of these a "fail-safe" method. Fentanyl pharmacokinetics after epidural and intrathecal administration have been discussed widely but with little rigorous data.

The development of a transdermal preparation of fentanyl base presents an interesting innovation in noninvasive dosage forms. The pharmacokinetics after this form of administration are complex (see, for example, [18, 30, 92, 13, 23, 46, 62, 64, 90, 24]), and are given in a separate chapter (see K. Gourlay and L. E. Mather, this volume).

Pharmacokinetic Philosophy

To many prescribers and/or administrators of drugs, the pharmacokinetic properties of a drug are no more interesting than its melting point! This, in part, derives from the way that pharmacokinetics is commonly taught – as a mathematical matter. For pharmacokinetics to have widespread clinical relevance, physiological and anatomical aspects need to be considered also. In this chapter the pharmacokinetics of fentanyl are reviewed with emphasis on the physiological and anatomical perspective. Although pharmacokinetics is the study of the time course of drug concentrations in various biofluids and tissues, it remains somewhat esoteric without consideration of the time course of the effects caused by the drug! Thus, the issue of drug-receptor kinetics, which also needs to be considered, is addressed en passant by pharmacokinetic-pharmacodynamic modelling techniques.

The fundamental pharmacokinetic properties of any drug are the rate and extent of distribution in the body and the rate and route(s) of elimination from the body. Because of the relative ease of experimentation, these are more often studied using tracer kinetic principles (apparent distribution volumes, microscopic rate constants and clearances) than using anatomical-physiological principles (regional blood flow, regional drug flux and/or clearance and regional drug partition coefficients). The other fundamental properties, half-life/lives and mean transit time(s), can be derived from these. If the drug has to be introduced into the body by some process involving absorption, then the rate(s) and extent of absorption become of interest also. Mathematical formulae for the calculation of pharmacokinetic parameters are widely available (e.g. [85, 93]) and are not discussed further in this chapter.

Fentanyl Pharmacokinetics

Fentanyl pharmacokinetics have been reviewed comprehensively, both in the English [58, 5] and German languages [47]. An important point made in the first comprehensive review [58] concerned the unusually large variability in results reported by different investigators: the potential significance of this variability has since been addressed by others [66]. The present review seeks to

a) update the previous reviews, and
b) rationalize the previously reported variability in fentanyl pharmacokinetics. Both the traditional empirical and contemporary anatomical-physiological approaches are used.

Relevance of the Physicochemical Properties of Fentanyl

The chemistry of fentanyl [*N*-(1-phenyl-4-piperidyl)-propionanilide] is dominated by three structural features: a large hydrocarbon mass giving lipophilic characteristics, an amide functional group giving a ready metabolic site, and a piperidine ring tertiary amine functional group (pK_a 8.43) [60] giving another ready metabolic site. Fentanyl is made water soluble through conjugate acid formation with citric acid where the base comprises 63.65 % of the formula weight. The amine group results in fentanyl being mostly in the ionized state at all values of physiological pH. Small changes in pH around the pH of plasma will make relatively large differences to the fraction ionized and, by inference, to the lipid solubility and therefore to the distribution (and potentially to the pharmacological action) of fentanyl. For example, in blood of pH 7.4 fentanyl is 9 % unionized, in acidotic blood (pH 7.1) fentanyl is 4 % unionized, and in alkalotic blood (pH 7.7) fentanyl is 16 % unionized.

Whether there is a difference in pharmacological activity resulting from such differences is difficult to determine, as other relevant changes also occur, e.g., parallel changes in plasma binding. Nevertheless, the ion-trapping of ionized fentanyl occurs in the highly acidic gastric juice, and its subsequent gastric reabsorption has been one explanation for the "secondary peak" phenomenon [73, 72]. Fentanyl does not contain a chiral center and is therefore not subject to additional pharmacokinetic and pharmacodynamic complications by having enantiomers (optical isomers).

Relevance of the Methods of Fentanyl Analysis

It has been suggested that the assay method of fentanyl analysis was implicated in the variability in fentanyl pharmacokinetics reported between various investigators [58]. Assay techniques have improved over the last decade. With respect to contemporary methods of fentanyl assay, gas-liquid chromatography (GLC) and high performance liquid chromatography (HPLC) can be used after solvent extraction to determine drug concentrations in any biofluid or tissue but radioimmunoassay (RIA) is generally restricted to noncellular preparations. The problems for all methods are those related to sensitivity because blood fentanyl concentrations of less than 0.5 ng/ml need accurate quantitation.

Recent GLC assays using solvent extraction preceding chromatography with nitrogen-phosphorus detection (NPD) or mass spectrometry (MS) are capable of measuring fentanyl to about 0.1 ng/ml of biological fluid with a reproducibility of 5%–10% (e.g. [43, 8, 90]). Recent RIAs are capable of similar performance [99]. Conventional HPLC with ultraviolet detection [44] is not as sensitive as GLC-NPD or GLC-MS. The illegal use of fentanyl in the horse racing industry and elsewhere has led to the development of a variety of rapid analyses for fentanyl but most would seem to lack the sensitivity required for detailed human pharmacokinetic investigations (e.g. [79, 17, 96]).

Much of the variability in assay results can be traced to the extraction processes (solvent interface and adsorption phenomena) so that minimizing the number of extractions (used to clean up the sample and concentrate the analyte) improves the reproducibility. The choice of assay technique should be based upon the demonstrated specificity of the method and on the type of biological sample to be assayed. GLC and HPLC are almost always specific or can be made so by choice of conditions; RIA may differ in performance between laboratories due to differences in antisera. The finding of Schüttler and White [74] that the order of addition of reagents in the assay by RIA kit caused a 29%–76% overestimate of fentanyl concentrations raises an additional concern over the widespread use of this method and the fentanyl concentration data acquired with this method.

Relevance of the Methods of Pharmacokinetic Analysis

Fentanyl, administered as the citrate salt, is frequently used intravenously as an intraoperative analgesic agent and as a postoperative analgesic agent, often with a patient-controlled analgesia (PCA) apparatus. Because of a short duration of action of single doses, fentanyl was originally thought to have a short half-life in the body. This notion persisted for many years but comprehensive pharmacokinetic studies have now provided data to the contrary. In the majority of studies in humans, fentanyl pharmacokinetic data have been calculated from coefficients and exponents of polyexponential decay equations fitted to fentanyl concentrations in a "representative body fluid" (blood, plasma or serum from a peripheral artery or vein). From these, the mean total body clearance (TBCl), initial (V) and total (Vss) apparent volumes of distribution, and half-lives ($T_{1/2}$) have been derived. A representative selection of the results of this approach is given in Fig. 1 and Table 1.

Undoubtedly, some of the variability in reported pharmacokinetics of fentanyl derives from the samples regarded as "representative samples" and assayed. Fentanyl is commonly studied intraoperatively when used as part of the anesthetic regimen, e.g., in patients undergoing cardiac bypass surgery. These patients often have an arterial cannula inserted and this has been used for sampling blood for fentanyl assays. When it has been used for postoperative analgesia or in volunteer subjects, peripheral venous blood samples for fentanyl assay have usually been collected.

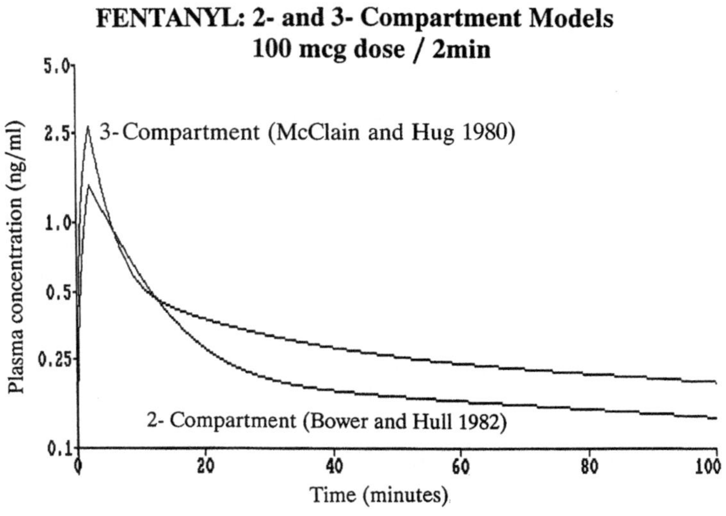

Fig. 1. The time course of plasma fentanyl concentrations (logarithmic scale) predicted from two reported pharmacokinetic studies. Study 1 used arterial drug concentrations, a radioactive label assay and a three compartment open model [59]; Study 2 used arm venous drug concentrations, a radioimmunoassay and a two compartment model

Table 1. The pharmacokinetic properties of fentanyl from three representative literature sources

	McClain and Hug (1980)[a]	Varvel et al. (1989)[b]	Bower and Hull (1982)[c]
Rapid $T_{1/2}$ (min)	1.65 (0.22)	1.35 (0.77)	NR
Intermedial $T_{1/2}$ (min)	12.7 (3.1)	24.7 (27.7)	NA
Slow $T_{1/2}$ (min)	241 (66)	428 (239)	185 (70)
Vc (l)	26.6 (9.8)	15.9 (8.9)	60 (18)
Vss (l)	311 (36)	398 (163)	335 (143)
TBCl (l/min)	0.88 (0.17)	0.77 (0.33)	1.53 (0.25)

NR, not reported; NA, not applicable; $T_{1/2}$, half-life; Vc, initial dilution volume; Vss, total apparent volume of distribution; TBCl, mean total body clearance

[a] Arterial plasma, 3H-assay, triexponential curve fit, healthy volunteers

[b] Arterial serum, GLC-MS assay, triexponential curve fit, surgical patients

[c] Venous plasma, RIA, biexponential curve fit, healthy volunteers.

It is important to note the details of the blood sampling protocol for a number of reasons:

1. If drug is being added to, or removed from, the body there will be regional blood drug concentration gradients. Arterial concentrations are those entering and venous concentrations are those leaving a region (except for the lungs in both cases). Venous concentrations therefore reflect the distribution of the drug in the region being drained: they are therefore "damped" and diluted during this additional transit through the tissues. Mixed venous blood raises the additional concern of blood "streaming" contributing to inhomogeneous drug concentrations but this is hard to verify in practice. The outcome is that arterial concentration-time data are often best fit by a three-exponential equation (leading to a three-compartment model of drug disposition when compartment models were more fashionable) and venous data by a two-exponential equation (and a two-compartment model). The pharmacokinetic parameters of each model are generally not interchangable: this most forcefully applies to the initial dilution volume and to micro rate constants. The sample source needs to be clearly defined.
2. The frequency of sampling also influences the number of terms in the exponential equation: the more data during the periods of rapid change, the more likely that a three-exponential equation will better fit the data.
3. The duration of sampling also plays a critical role. The longer the duration of sampling, the more likely the drug washout from poorly perfused tissues or drug elimination will be determined accurately by the terminal slope measured. This is also applied to studies performed during drug infusion so that TBCl can be calculated without including drug loss by distribution.

4. Factors influencing tissue blood flow (e.g. hepatic, renal) or the distribution of tissue blood flow (e.g., skin: muscle ratio) can influence the measured pharmacokinetics, e.g., general anesthesia and neural blockade, and thereby influence the time course of blood drug concentrations. This is a major potential reason for secondary blood drug concentration peaks (see [71]).
5. Different experimental designs, viz., bolus versus infusion, may maximize one or the other element of perfusion (bolus design) against diffusion (infusion design) in determining the extent of blood : tissue equilibration during washin and washout and, thereby, the pharmacokinetic parameters. Thus, there should be no surprise that two-compartment models are suggested by some experiments and three-compartment models by others: the choice of a pharmacokinetic model depends to a large extent upon the experimental design and its value depends upon the purpose of creating the model and of the quality of the data used in its construction.

No matter what method is used for the pharmacokinetic analysis the dose must be known accurately. While it should be safe to assume that the dose has been correct and that the difference between fentanyl and fentanyl citrate has been taken into account, such optimism is not necessarily well-placed. For example, almost 70 % of fentanyl added to cardiopulmonary bypass equipment can be lost [36, 41]. Although many drugs are adsorbed by medical plastics and/or glass in drug administration systems [89], it has been found that fentanyl losses at room temperature in 0.9 % saline or 5 % dextrose in glass or plastic containers for ODAC-PCA (On-Demand Analgesic Computer, Janssen Scientific Instruments Beerse) were generally insignificant (<5 %) during storage for 48 h [42]. However, studies of fentanyl losses into the plastics of syringes and/or other apparatus used in pharmacokinetic analysis [87] have not been reported. Other potential problems are whether the accuracy of dilutions of injections take into account any overage of volume supplied in containers of fluid for injection and whether blood samples for analysis are contaminated by being drawn through the same cannula used for drug injection.

Relevance of Intravascular Distribution of Fentanyl

The choice of the biofluid for pharmacokinetic analysis often depends on analytical considerations, but it should depend on the use to which the data will be put. If the purpose is comparative, then plasma or serum concentrations will usually suffice, but if the purpose is absolute, e.g., calculation of physiological mass balance, blood concentrations are usually required. If the drug equilibrates quickly and distributes uniformly between blood cells and plasma, then blood and plasma are equivalent in usefulness. The common practice of measuring drug concentrations in plasma and then converting them to "blood concentrations" by dividing by "the blood : plasma concentration ratio" previously determined in vitro may be erroneous if the ratio is concentration-dependent, acid-base sensitive, or subject to other experimental variables in vivo that are not completely accounted for in vitro.

Binding of fentanyl to blood cells and to plasma proteins has been discussed in previous reviews and new information of significance has not been produced since these reviews. In brief, systematic studies [35, 60, 59, 51] have shown that the partitioning of fentanyl into erythrocytes is rapid and the blood : plasma partition coefficient (approximately 1.0) is not significantly affected by hematocrit, pH, or a range of (total) drug concentrations. Because plasma protein binding increases with pH (from approximately 85 % at pH 7.4 to approximately 90 % at pH 8.0) it is rationalized that parallel changes occur in erythrocyte binding so that the blood : plasma partition coefficient does not change with pH. Although it is tempting to speculate about fentanyl distribution between blood and tissues as a function of pH and binding, it is a difficult issue to resolve because of the occurrence of other changes. For example, it has been shown that fentanyl blood and brain concentration were greater in dogs that were hypocarbic than in those that were either normocarbic or hypercarbic [1]. However, the concurrent effects of carbon dioxide on regional blood flow make it difficult to explain the results by one mechanism.

A number of proteins in plasma are involved in fentanyl binding. As is often found for drugs that are weak organic bases, the highest affinity for fentanyl occurs by binding with alpha$_1$-acid glycoprotein. However, because alpha$_1$-acid glycoprotein is an acute phase reactant protein, physiological and pathophysiological states that influence the concentration of this protein (for example, early neonatal age → decreased concentration; trauma → increased concentration) could have an exaggerated influence on the pharmacokinetics of fentanyl, although this has not been demonstrated experimentally. A transplacental gradient of binding proteins is the presumed mechanism for the transplacental gradient of fentanyl being maintained at a value <1.0 (e.g. [91, 61].

Relevance of Extravascular Distribution of Fentanyl

For most drugs the blood is only a means of transport to sites of action, distribution and clearance: this is also the case for fentanyl. Much misunderstanding in pharmacokinetics and pharmacodynamics can be traced to the failure of investigators to think in terms of regional anatomy and physiology and this, too, applies in studies of fentanyl. The expectation that drug concentrations in peripheral blood will predict drug effects in the CNS has led to a number of methods for tailoring intravenous drug administration rates based upon pharmacokinetic data. A number of papers testing such methods based upon the observed and predicted concentrations of fentanyl and other opioids have now been published (e.g. [3, 6, 55, 54, 65]). The methodology is successful in predicting group average values but, although some valuable starting points have been achieved, the more serious problem of predicting individual values by way of population pharmacokinetics is in need of further attention.

Relevance of Receptor Kinetics to Blood Fentanyl Concentrations

Fentanyl, like its congeners sufentanil and alfentanil, is often chosen for a rapid onset of pharmacological action which is believed to be a result of its lipophilicity. From EEG signal changes and combined pharmacokinetic-pharmacodynamic modelling, a mean blood-receptor equilibration half-life of approximately 5 min has been found for both fentanyl and sufentanil. However, a value of approximately 1 min, found for the less lipophilic alfentanil under the same experimental conditions [76, 77, 15, 16], indicates that lipophilicity alone does not determine that rate of onset of action. The rate of onset is a function of two properties: the diffusible drug concentration in blood (determined by the products of the drug concentration and the unbound and ionized fractions) and the blood : tissue partition coefficients (that determine the capacity for tissues to fill with drug) [35]. Therefore, a high diffusible fraction (Table 2) is a very important factor. Rapid receptor association and dissociation of fentanyl as measured in vitro has been reported [10] and this, when coupled with the high lipophilicity, is a necessary condition for blood concentrations to reflect receptor concentrations, and therefore pharmacological effect.

When fentanyl is used intraoperatively as an analgesic agent the target blood drug concentrations would appear to range from approximately 3- to >20 ng/ml, depending on other medication used (e.g., nitrous oxide), the criteria used for defining the target, and the severity of the stimulus (Table 3). When used postoperatively with PCA apparatus, a mean "minimum effective blood concentration" (the average blood concentration at which patients activated their apparatus) in 30 patients during a mean of 50 h after lower abdominal surgery was found to be 0.6 ng/ml (range 0.23–1.18 ng/ml) [25]. In

Table 2. Some relevant physicochemical properties of fentanyl and comparisons with some other important opioid agonists

	pK_a [a]	Octanol Coefficient [b]	% Base [c]	% Free [d]	% Diffusible fraction [e]
Fentanyl	8.4	11 220	9	16	1
Pethidine	8.7	525	7	60	4
Alfentanil	6.5	145	89	9	8

[a] Dissociation constant of conjugate acid form
[b] Octanol: water partition coefficient of base
[c] Percentage in unionized form according to the Henderson-Hasselbalch equation
[d] Percentage unbound in plasma (typical value in adult human plasma)
[e] Product of % Base and % Free

Table 3. The relationship between fentanyl plasma concentration and effect

Concentration (ng/ml)	Effect
10 (approximately) –30	Unconsciousness
10–20	Responsiveness suppressed during surgery
5–10	EEG slowing
3+	Intraoperative analgesia
1.5–4	50 % depression in CO_2 response curve
0.7–1.2	Postoperative analgesia (mean values)
<0.7	Insignificant respiratory effects

a different study by other investigators, a median value of 1.2 ng/ml (fentanyl serum concentration, range 0.2–8.0 ng/ml) was found [53].

There is no uniform opinion as to whether there really is a "minimum effective blood concentration" of opioids in this setting [48] as other work has shown the value may depend upon other factors including the dosage prescription used (demand bolus size and concurrent background infusion) and the duration (development of tolerance?). The argument in favor of the proposition of a "minimum effective blood concentration" of fentanyl is based upon the greater reproducibility of values for individual patients than between patients (as has now been demonstrated for a variety of opioids). The argument against is based upon the lack of a clear-cut threshold minimum drug concentration for effect. The arguments must be balanced by recognizing the highly subjective nature of the endpoint and of confounding features such as changing level of stimulus due to the wound and changing level of effect due to perioperative drug use and endogenous opioid control and to acute tolerance to the drug being evaluated.

The expectation that blood concentrations will reflect receptor concentrations (and therefore pharmacological effect) has produced a sizeable literature on pharmacokinetic-pharmacodynamic modelling based on the time-course of drug concentration in a hypothetical receptor-containing "effect-causing" compartment of the body [29]. This elegant approach, which was developed to offset the limitations of less-than-ideal experimental designs attainable in humans, provides two parameters from such an analysis – the rate constant (or the half-life) of drug equilibration and the lag time for effect [19]. The principal difficulty with this work as applied to opioids [78, 76, 75] is that the pharmacological effect chosen to be modelled (alterations to the EEG power spectrum, see [33]) has neither been shown to be a clinically relevant effect in itself nor a specific effect of opioid receptor stimulation.

Relevance of Fentanyl Regional Kinetics

Regional pharmacokinetics involves study of the time course of drug concentrations in affluent and effluent blood of particular regions and tissues of the body. Much recent attention has been directed towards the pulmonary first-pass extraction of drugs, and rightly so, because the lungs are the first region encountered by a drug admitted to the venous blood. There is considerable evidence that the lungs act to impede the transit of most drugs, including fentanyl and other opioid analgesics. For these agents, the lung "uptake" (which is rather ill-defined pharmacokinetically) or first-pass extraction increases with the lipophilicity of the drugs, e.g., approximately 70 %–85 % extraction of fentanyl (compared to approximately 50 %–65 % of meperidine and alfentanil and approximately <10 % of morphine [68, 84]. This effect takes on an important role when drugs are admitted rapidly into the blood and causes arterial concentrations to be attenuated in magnitude and spread in time, thereby moderating their effects on vital organ systems. However, "pulmonary uptake" is not synonymous with metabolic clearance in the lungs. Unless there is metabolic clearance, drug lost to the lungs is regained as the initial concentration gradient from blood to tissue is dissipated. Most reports contain only the first pass (positive) extraction, i.e., usually over only 1 min or so after IV bolus administration, and leave the suggestion that this may be clearance; they do not indicate the extended time-course showing negative extraction (release back into the blood). This is not to say that drugs are not cleared by the lungs. They may be so cleared, but apart from volatile or gaseous substances, there are relatively few examples in which the lungs have been proven major sites of drug clearance in vivo. That the uptake is due to reasonably selective binding is suggested by the observation that fentanyl pulmonary uptake was less in patients who had been treated with the lipophilic basic amine propranolol than in those who had not [67].

Using anatomical reference points, application of the Law of Conservation of Matter to each regional drug (and/or metabolite) concentration gradient and blood flow allows the rate of drug distribution (regional net drug flux) and regional clearance to be determined. The time integral of the net flux gives the regional net drug mass which, if divided by the organ mass, gives the regional drug concentration. From the total body and the measured regional fluxes and clearances of a drug and metabolites, the total fate may be determined [88]. The benefits of this methodology are that the effects of physiological or pathological perturbations on total body and regional drug mass balance can be assessed in a nondestructive manner and that both drug washin and drug washout experimental designs can be used.

The regional pharmacokinetics of fentanyl have not yet been systematically investigated, but some preliminary data on its regional kinetics in intact sheep (Mather et al., work in progress) are presented. Figure 2 shows regional net fluxes of fentanyl derived from its concentrations in blood samples taken simultaneously from the ascending aorta, pulmonary artery, hepatic and renal veins and inferior vena cava (distal to the kidneys) after a bolus iv injection using the methodology of Upton et al. [88]. It can be seen that during the first 10–15 min the lungs are releasing fentanyl distributed there from its initial uptake (negative flux), the liver and hindquarters are taking up substantial amounts of fentanyl (positive flux), and the kidneys are taking up

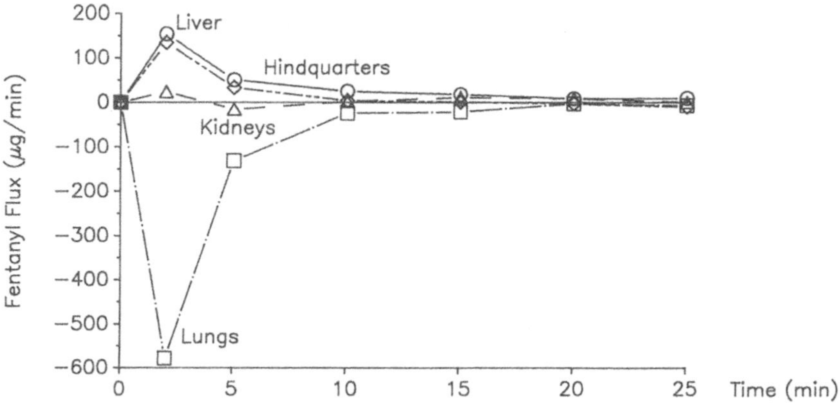

Fig. 2. Preliminary data on the regional pharmacokinetics of fentanyl in the chronically cannulated intact sheep. The net fluxes between blood and lungs, liver, kidneys, and hindquarters (a representative nonvisceral region) are shown after an intravenous bolus dose of 2500 μg fentanyl citrate. Positive flux is net uptake; negative flux is net release

only a very small amount of fentanyl. By 4 h (Fig. 3), the mass of fentanyl released by the lungs is approximately equal to the total dose injected, the liver has removed approximately 60 % of the dose, the kidneys have removed approximately 20 % of the dose, and the hindquarters still contain approximately 13 % of the dose. By later time points, inferior vena cava blood fentanyl concentrations exceed those in arterial blood, indicating a net

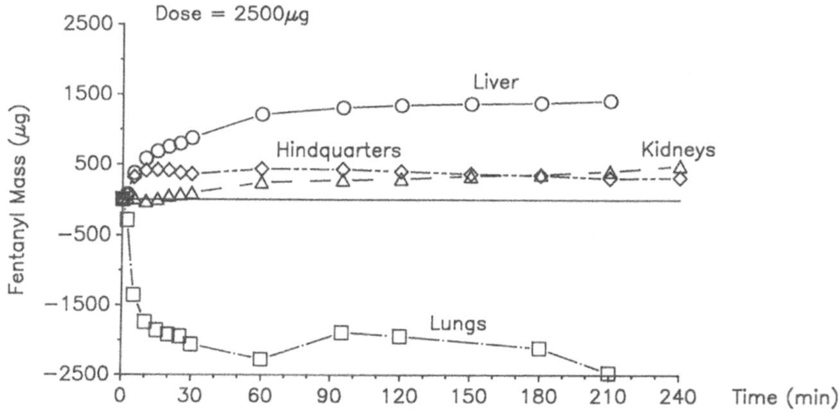

Fig. 3. Preliminary data on the regional pharmacokinetics of fentanyl in the chronically cannulated intact sheep. The mass of fentanyl in the lungs, liver, kidneys, and hindquarters (a representative nonvisceral region) are shown after an intravenous bolus dose of 2500 μg fentanyl citrate. The negative mass in the lungs represents the amount released by the tissue. The positive mass represents the amount that has been delivered to the tissue by the arterial blood that has not been removed by the venous blood. For the liver and kidneys, this is assumed to represent the amount cleared; for the hindquarters it is assumed to be the amount distributed

washout of drug from the hindquarter region drained by the inferior vena cava. It is interesting to note that there is also evidence of secondary blood fentanyl concentration peaks occurring in this study (Fig. 4). The sheep, as a ruminant, has a large volume of acidic rumen (approximately 4 l) and mention has been made previously of the propensity for gastric ion-trapping and subsequent gastric reabsorption of basic drugs in this species [69, 56]. However, the secondary peak cannot be traced to fentanyl release via hepatic venous plasma for subsequent recirculation; instead, the peak would appear to be more associated with changed concentration in nonvisceral mass (as represented in this experiment by the hindquarters), which is muscle, fat etc.

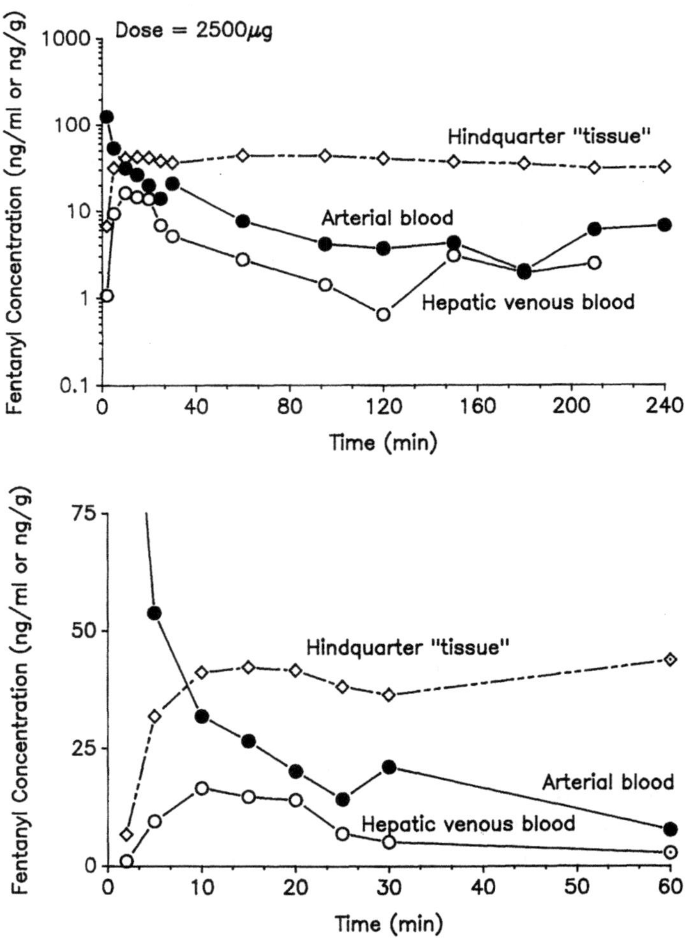

Fig. 4. Preliminary data on the regional pharmacokinetics of fentanyl in the chronically cannulated intact sheep. Fentanyl concentrations in arterial and hepatic venous blood are shown together with the derived "hindquarter tissue" concentration. *The lower graph* shows the same data on a time-expanded scale

In Fig. 5, the uptake and release of fentanyl into the brain of the sheep is shown in comparison to that of morphine when the two substances are injected into the right atrium mixed together. From this it is clear that in this study the rate of uptake of morphine into brain tissue was slightly greater than that of fentanyl, which is a different conclusion to that from the classical work of Herz and Teschemacher [27]. It is therefore concluded that the most important factor in the brain uptake and release of such substances is the drug concentration gradient between blood and tissue. If the rate of administration is rapid, then this gradient will be high and therefore the rate of uptake will be rapid. As the concentration gradient falls due to continued drug distribution and clearance, the rate of release will be greater for substances having the ability to transfer readily down a now very small concentration gradient. Therefore, morphine, being less lipophilic than fentanyl is released more slowly. This conclusion has also been reached by Lehmann [47] from comparison of studies by others [1, 63] in which blood and brain tissues were sampled directly.

The liver and, to a lesser extent, the kidneys, are the principal regions of fentanyl clearance although other regions may contribute as well, particularly in species other than humans [50]. The role of the (sheep) liver is clear also from the data in Figs. 2, 3. Another study potentially relevant to fentanyl regional pharmacokinetics showed that pethidine was extracted by the liver and kidneys but not by the lungs or gut in sheep [56, 57]. However, for pethidine, the discrepancy between the total body and the summed visceral clearances indicated that sundry nonvisceral regions also must be involved to a major extent. Cannulation of the venous drainage of the sheep hindquarters showed that mean steady-state pethidine extraction ratio was 0.4 and the corresponding clearance was approximately 0.8 l/min (20% of total body clearance). Similar extraction ratios would occur in regions of similar anatomical composition such as the forequarters and chest wall, with clearances in proportion to the regional blood flows. In this case, an appreciable portion of the total body clearance was unexpectedly accounted for by nonvisceral clearance, this presumably being explained on teleological grounds in relation to the natural diet of the sheep. Study of the extrahepatic metabolism of fentanyl has been performed in vitro [47] but investigation of its importance in vivo still remains for systematic studies.

Regional pharmacokinetic data gathered from destructive methods in laboratory rodents have been reported for fentanyl by a number of investigators [28, 34, 49, 72, 9]. Autoradiographic studies using a drug washout design have shown clearly that fentanyl reaches high concentrations first in the lungs, the CNS and the myocardium. This is followed by redistribution to the kidneys, liver, gut and stomach contents, then to skeletal muscle, bone marrow and salivary glands. Recent studies using a drug washin design in rats have allowed redetermination of the regional tissue : blood partition coefficients and have applied these values to the stimulation of the time-course of fentanyl tissue concentrations in humans [9]. Every tissue analysed had partition coefficient >1. Of particular note were the high values

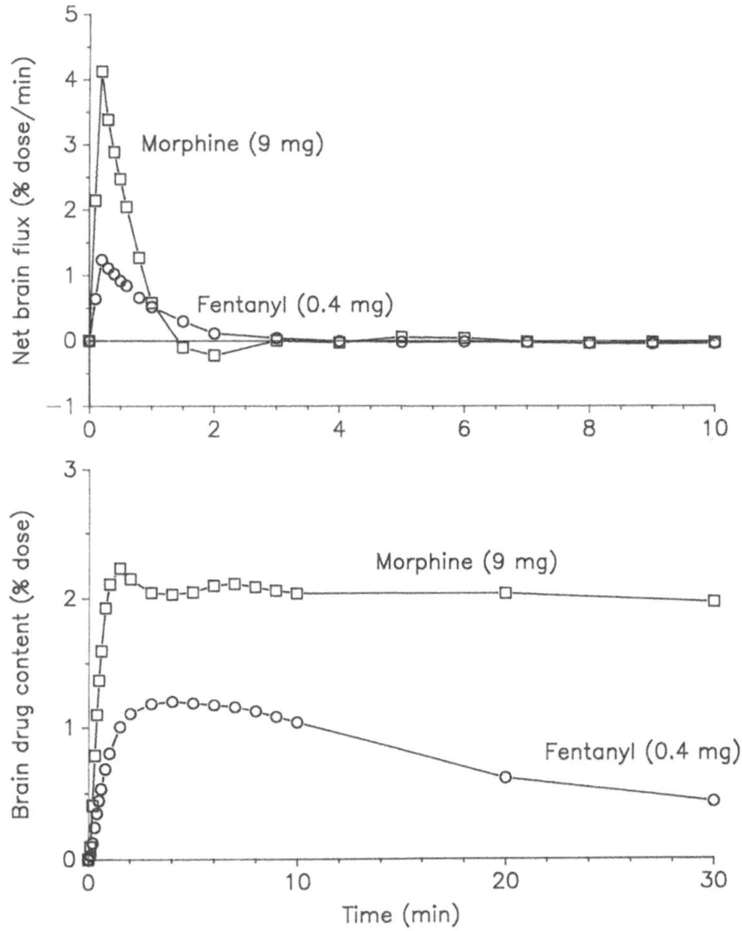

Fig. 5. Preliminary data on the regional pharmacokinetics of fentanyl in the chronically cannulated intact sheep. *Top:* the net fluxes between blood and brain are shown after a pre-mixed intravenous bolus dose of 0.4 mg fentanyl citrate plus 9 mg morphine sulphate pentahydrate. Positive flux is net uptake, negative flux is net release. *Bottom:* the masses of fentanyl and morphine in the brain are shown. The positive mass represents the amount that has been delivered to the tissue by the arterial blood that has not been removed by the venous blood

reported for lungs (15.3) and for fat (30.2). Unfortunately a value for skin, which also comprises a large regional body mass (and a high potential for drug uptake and release), was not determined.

It is emphasized that pharmacokinetic models formed by sampling only systemic blood can be used only to predict systemic blood concentrations. However, sampling regional blood and or tissue drug concentrations allows pharmacokinetic modelling which preserves anatomical and physiological veracity and insight that cannot be gained by studying systemic pharmacokinetics alone. Unfortunately, the difficulty of performing such experiment makes them inaccessible for most researchers.

Relevance of other Drugs to Fentanyl Pharmacokinetics

Another relevant physiological assumption in pharmacokinetics is that of stationarity i.e., the constancy in time of "the system" being studied. This is necessary so that time-averaged apparent volumes of distribution and total body clearances can be calculated. Violation of this assumption most commonly occurs in the perioperative period – a popular time for pharmacokinetic studies of opioid analgesics. Study designs often involve studies commencing shortly after the induction of anesthesia with the continuation of blood sampling for drug analysis through the perioperative course. The "appropriate" pharmacokinetic model is applied to the resultant serial blood concentration-time data if the drug's kinetics were the same throughout the entire perioperative period.

It is now well known that anesthesia, surgery, acid-base balance, etc., may each markedly influence pharmacokinetics. It therefore must be clear that the results of such a time-averaged pharmacokinetic analysis may bear no relationship to the "true pharmacokinetics" of any individual period. Indeed it is probable that the dominant effect may be that of the anesthetic agents or anesthesia on drug distribution and clearance [70]. It has not been possible to dissect out the individual effects in studies of fentanyl although it is known that different anesthetic regimens alter fentanyl systemic kinetics [52, 47] in vivo and its pattern of metabolism in vitro [50, 47]. By systematic regional pharmacokinetic studies in chronically catheterized sheep it has been shown that anesthesia alone with either intravenous or inhalation agents will increase by approximately 100 % arterial blood steady-state concentrations of drugs such as pethidine, which recover to baseline values 3–6 h after anesthesia. This has been shown to be caused by the combined effects of anesthesia upon regional blood flow and pethidine clearance, and to decreases in the apparent volume of distribution of pethidine [57]. Such drug interactions would seem to be an inevitable consequence of anesthesia [70]. While similar regional kinetic effects undoubtedly occur with fentanyl, to date systematic observations on the effects of anesthesia have only been made for fentanyl systemic kinetics [47].

By considering all the perioperative drug concentrations-time data as a continuum, a pharmacokinetic model can be produced but the value of such a model is dubious as it combines the pharmacokinetic properties of the drug with the physiological perturbations of the perioperative period. Despite this limitation, there are many reports of fentanyl pharmacokinetics in the perioperative period that are of help in designing dosage regimens for producing target blood drug concentrations (e.g. [18, 32, 37]). Under strictly controlled conditions, it may be possible to reproduce a dose-drug blood concentration relationship, but this will not demonstrate the drug's "true pharmacokinetics". Therefore, to decide from such data on a "preferred pharmacokinetic model" (e.g. [32]) under such multifactorial conditions seems to be overly optimistic.

Relevance of Route of Administration to Fentanyl Pharmacokinetics

Intramuscular injections of fentanyl would be expected to produce erratic blood drug concentrations due to unpredictable and erratic systemic absorption of fentanyl and, indeed, this has been found. In different studies, mean maximum plasma fentanyl concentrations of 0.6–0.8 ng/ml were found to result from IM injection of approximately 1.5–2 μg/kg [39, 47]. The erratic blood concentration response is not surprising. With such a lipophilic substance, apart from differences between subjects in systemic kinetics, small differences in the method of intramuscular injection could result in the fentanyl being deposited in muscle body or in fatty tissues for which the affinity would differ and from which the rate of absorption would differ markedly.

Oral fentanyl has little place in pain pharmacotherapy because of high hepatosplanchnic clearance. When administered to anesthetized patients by nasogastric tube at a dose of 4 μg/kg, plasma fentanyl concentrations were found to be very irregular, with high interpatient variability and a mean maximum of approximately 0.2 ng/ml 5 h after administration [47]. An oral bioavailability of only 1.5 % was found in the rat [72].

Recent use has been made of the high lipid solubility of fentanyl base in the oral-buccal administration of fentanyl using experimental "lollipop" and sublingual dosage forms [82, 83, 94]. Inhalation of nebulized fentanyl produces sustained blood drug concentrations consistent with about 10 % bioavailability [97]. It would be expected that swallowed fentanyl from all of these routes would contribute little to the blood drug concentrations, making each of these a fail-safe method.

Not infrequently, the blood and CSF concentrations of analgesic drugs after epidural or intrathecal administration are measured to determine the relevant pharmacokinetics. However, without knowledge of the concurrent intravascular pharmacokinetics this approach cannot yield anything but simple descriptive and/or comparative parameters such as the maximum drug concentration and the time at which it occurs. Even the time course of absorption is impossible to determine accurately because of the influence of drug partitioning and subsequent slow absorption from epidural fat. Because of the broad similarity of physicochemical properties, it would be expected that fentanyl would be systemically absorbed in a manner similar to bupivacaine [86, 11]. Thus it would be expected that, despite the rapidity with which peak arterial blood drug concentrations are obtained (<20 min) [39, 2], the absorption profile would be biphasic. For bupivacaine approximately one-third of the dose is absorbed rapidly with a half-life of <30 min, and the remainder with a half-life of 4–8 h, corresponding to the absorption from fatty structures. The corollary of the lipophilicity of fentanyl is that its systemic absorption and local deposition allows minimal cephalad drug transport in CSF and thereby reduces the likelihood of its causing late-onset respiratory depression.

Sometimes the time-course of a drug in CSF has been used to calculate the drug's CSF clearance and apparent CSF volume of distribution. Because the sampled CSF is not well-mixed and homogeneous with respect to drug concentration these calculations are invalid. It is plain that the concentration in CSF will depend upon the rate of mixing and the site of sampling. It is valid to compare the time-course of substances injected together so that differences between agents can be determined. From this approach, the influence of drug polarity on drug kinetics, for example, has been studied [22]. In another study, the passage of fentanyl into CSF and its cephalad migration was studied after intravenous and lumbar epidural administration [26]. It was concluded that there was insignificant transfer of fentanyl to lumbar CSF after intravenous administration but facile and significant transfer after epidural administration. Fentanyl interaction with spinal cord opioid receptors would be of little consequence in providing analgesia after intravenous administration. Fentanyl blood concentrations were essentially undetectable and fentanyl cervical CSF concentrations were insignificant in patients after lumbar epidural administration. Therefore, stimulation of opioid receptors in the brain after epidural administration would be of little consequence in providing analgesia.

Fentanyl blood concentrations after epidural administration have been discussed widely (e.g. [47, 39, 45]) but there are not sufficient data from reliable fentanyl assays from which the absorption kinetics of fentanyl can be determined reliably as, for example, has been done for pethidine [21]. In one of very few quantitative pharmacokinetic studies, about 1%–3% fentanyl availability to the CSF has been shown after epidural administration in the goat [4].

Relevance of Fentanyl Pharmacokinetics to Clinical Practice

Fentanyl has a high clearance but after single or infrequent doses, its duration of action is terminated by redistribution [34]. The high lipid solubility of fentanyl helps it to have both a rapid onset due to facile CNS penetration and a brief duration of action as the drug continues to move down the concentration gradient to muscle and to fat [51, 47, 9]. Drug is readily removed from blood (so that the measured "clearance" is high (Table 3), but slow removal from the fat pools causes the plasma half-life to become longer than the duration of action. As explained above, determination of the true plasma clearance and half-life of fentanyl is difficult because of lack of sensitivity of the assays to the low blood concentrations occurring after normal doses. As fentanyl assays have become more sensitive, it is possible to see more of the washout from the body, and that this takes place at a slower rate than originally believed. Because the half-life is long, accumulation can occur if pain is treated with frequently repeated doses. Respiratory depression may then become a problem [7]. The problem of understanding strategies for drug delivery to various patient groups then becomes important and is facilitated by knowledge of drug disposition in different conditions.

In various studies, age and size of patient have been considered covariables of pharmacokinetic parameters. Within one group of male patients (ASA grades I–III), neither age nor body weight were related to the TBCl calculated from the ratio of the fentanyl infusion rate to (constant) mean arterial serum concentration over a range of 25, 50, 100 or 125 μg/h [30]. From a study of age as a determinant of fentanyl pharmacokinetics, Singleton et al. [81] reported that, after intravenous administration, only in the first 10 min of a 4 h study were plasma fentanyl concentrations greater in elderly (71–82 years) than in younger adults (18–41 years). As a consequence, it was reported that elderly patients had a volume of distribution that was an average of 60 % that of the younger patients but that the TBCl, mean residence time and $T_{1/2Z}$ did not differ between groups. If the brain uptake is related to the arterial-to-brain drug concentration gradient, then this discrepancy could make a large difference to the mass of drug in the brain and therefore to pharmacological effects. Reasons for the higher concentrations of fentanyl in elderly patients could include both an age-related reduction in cardiac output and an age-related reduction in fat-lean body distribution.

On the other end of the age spectrum, pharmacokinetics of fentanyl are not all clear. In patients aged 23–38 weeks being treated for patent *ductus arteriosus,* Collins et al. [14] found a similar apparent volume of distribution of fentanyl to that in adults (2.2–3.9 l/kg), but that the TBCl of fentanyl was only 2.4 ml/kg # min (compared to 12 ml/kg # min) and accordingly the $T_{1/2Z}$ was prolonged to 17.7 h (compared to 3–9 h). Others have not found the same outcome from similar experiments. For example, Singleton et al. [80] found the same apparent volume of distribution over a wide range of ages (3 months to 41 years) but that the TBCl was higher (31 ml/kg # min) in patients between 3 and 10 months so that the $T_{1/2Z}$ was shorter in this group. Johnson et al. [38] found that the $T_{1/2Z}$ was much the same in patients ranging in age from 1 day to 27 years but that Vss decreased. Khoentop et al. [40] found similar fentanyl pharmacokinetics in neonates to that commonly reported in adults. It is difficult to know from these studies whether the elimination efficiency of fentanyl is impaired in the young; at the same time, the plasma binding of opioids is usually lower in the younger age groups. Thus the mixed results could also indicate that the traditional method of comparison of values between different age groups (i.e., per kg body weight) may be in need of reconsideration as are the effect of pathology and or concurrent procedures on fentanyl disposition. Overriding all this is the problem of experimental design not being ideal or even uniform between studies. The conclusions tend to be based on poor data. As pointed out by Hudson [31], scientific enquiry and the ability to collect data have to be balanced against ethics and good medical practice, but this is no excuse for reporting poor data.

The vast majority of "clinical pharmacokinetic" studies of fentanyl to date have been performed with conventional methodology. Interpretation of mechanisms involved has not been possible because only a "black box" pharmacokinetic approach has been used. Improvements in clinical pharmacokinetic methodology are necessary! In order to make such improvements, relevant physiological methodology needs to be incorporated into pharmacokinetic methodology. For example, for evaluating the effects of age, it is necessary to reference against a suitable marker of maturation; what is a suitable marker – body weight, lean tissue mass, some biochemical marker ...? For that matter, how should dose be calculated?

Relevance of Pharmacokinetic Studies of Opioid Analgesic Agents

The information in this chapter provides a synopsis of fentanyl pharmacokinetics and pharmacodynamics. In again highlighting the issue of variability in fentanyl pharmacokinetics, it has become apparent that much of this can be ascribed to inconsistency in the many uncontrolled methodological variables.

The following variables potentially influence pharmacokinetic results:

1. Age, surgical procedures, pathology?
2. Patients or volunteers?
3. Dose, rate of administration, dose scaling factor?
4. Blood samples, site, frequency, duration?
5. Assay, specimen, sensitivity, reproducibility?
6. Pharmacokinetic methodology, art, science?
7. Results expression, raw data, derived values?

This list is not exhaustive. However, it is also clear that the use of anatomical and physiological principles can provide insight into the interpretation of fentanyl pharmacokinetics that is not revealed by traditional empirical methods.

References

1. Ainslie SG, Eisele JH, Corkill G (1979) Fentanyl concentrations in brain and serum during respiratory acid base changes in the dog. Anesthesiology 51: 293–297
2. Ahuja BR, Strunin L (1985) Respiratory effects of epidural fentanyl. Anaesthesia 40: 949–955
3. Alvis JM, Reves JG, Govier AV, Menkhans PG, Henling CE (1985) Computer assisted continuous infusions of fentanyl during cardiac anesthesia: comparison with a manual method. Anesthesiology 63: 41–49
4. Andersen HB, Christensen B, Findlay JW, Jansen JA (1986) Pharmacokinetics of intravenous, intrathecal and epidural morphine and fentanyl in the goat. Acta Anaesthesiol Scand 30: 393–399

5. Andrews CJH, Prys-Roberts C (1983) Fentanyl – a review. Clin Anaesthesiol 1:97–122
6. Ausems ME, Stanski DR, Hug CC Jr (1985) An evaluation of the accuracy of pharmacokinetic data for the computer assisted infusion of alfentanil. Br J Anaesth 57: 1217–1225
7. Bailey PL, Streisand JB, East KA, East TD, Alsern S, Hansen W, Posthuma EFM, Rozendaal FW, Pace NL, Stanley TH (1990) Differences in magnitude and duration of opioid induced respiratory depression and analgesia with fentanyl and sufentanil. Anesth Analg 70: 8–15
8. Bjorkman S, Stanski DR (1988) Simultaneous determination of fentanyl and alfentanil in rat tissues by capillary column gas chromatography. J Chromatogr 433: 95–104
9. Bjorkman S, Stanski DR, Verotta D, Harashima H (1990) Comparative tissue concentration profiles of fentanyl and alfentanil in humans predicted from tissue/blood partition data obtained in rats. Anesthesiology 72: 865–873
10. Boas RA, Villiger JW (1985) Clinical actions of fentanyl and buprenorphine. Br J Anaesth 57: 192–196
11. Bower S, Hull CJ (1982) Comperative pharmacokinetics of fentanyl and alfentanil. Br J Anaesth 54: 871–877
12. Burm A (1989) Clinical pharmacokinetics of epidural and spinal anaesthesia. Clin Pharmacokin 16: 283–311
13. Chauvin M, Strumza P, Guirimand F, Levron JC, Falson F, Duvaldestin P (1989) Concentrations plasmatiques de fentanyl administre par voie transdermique. Ann Fr Anesth Reanim 8 Suppl: R154
14. Collins C, Koren G, Crean P, Klein J, Roy WL, MacLeod SM (1985) Fentanyl pharmacokinetics and hemodynamic effects in preterm infants during ligation of patent ductus arteriosus. Anesth Analg 64: 1078–1080
15. Cooke JE, Scott JC (1986) Do sufentanil and fentanyl have the same pharmacodynamics? Anesthesiology 65: A552
16. Cooke JE, Scott JC (1987) Fentanyl vs. sufentanil: the same onset time. Anesthesiology 67: A393
17. Delbeke FT, Debackere (1989) ELISA detection of fentanyl in horse urine and plasma. J Vet Pharmacol Ther 12: 1–4
18. Duthie DJ, Rowbotham DJ, Wyld R, Henderson PD, Nimmo WS (1988) Plasma fentanyl concentrations during transdermal delivery of fentanyl to surgical patients. Br J Anaesth 60: 614–618
19. Duthie DJ, McLaren AD, Nimmo WS (1986) Pharmacokinetics of fentanyl during constant rate i.v. infusion for the relief of pain after surgery. Br J Anaesth 58: 950–956
20. Ebling WF, Lee EN, Stanski DR (1990) Understanding pharmacokinetics and pharmacodynamics through computer simulation: I. The comparative clinical profiles of fentanyl and alfentanil. Anesthesiology 72: 650–658
21. Glynn CJ, Mather LE, Cousins MJ, Graham JR, Wilson PR (1981) Peridural meperidine in man: analgetic response, pharmacokinetics and transmission into CSF. Anesthesiology 55: 520–526
22. Gourlay GK, Cherry DA, Plummer JL, Armstrong PJ, Cousins MJ (1987) The influence of drug polarity on the absorption of opioid drugs into CSF and subsequent cephalad migration following lumbar epidural administration: application to morphine and pethidine. Pain 31: 297–305
23. Gourlay GK, Kowalski SR, Plummer JL, Cherry DA, Gaukroger P, Cousins MJ (1989) The transdermal administration of fentanyl in the treatment of postoperative pain: pharmacokinetics and pharmacodynamic effects. Pain 37: 193–202
24. Gourlay GK, Kowalski SR, Plummer JL, Cherry DA, Szekely SM, Mather LE, Owen H, Cousins MJ (1990) The efficacy of transdermal fentanyl in the treatment of postoperative pain: a double blind comparison of fentanyl and placebo systems. Pain 40: 21–28

25. Gourlay GK, Kowalski SR, Plummer JL, Cousins MJ, Armstrong PJ (1988) Fentanyl blood concentration analgesic response relationship in the treatment of postoperative pain. Anesth Analg 67: 329–337
26. Gourlay GK, Murphy TM, Plummer JL, Kowalski SR, Cherry DA, Cousins MJ (1989) Pharmacokinetics of fentanyl in lumbar and cervical CSF following lumbar epidural and intravenous administration. Pain 38: 253–259
27. Herz A, Teschemacher H-J (1971) Activities and site of antinociceptive action of morphine-like kinetics of distribution following intravenous, intracerebral and intraventricular application. Adv Drug Res 6: 79–119
28. Hess R, Herz A, Friedel K (1972) Pharmacokinetics of fentanyl in rabbits in view of the importance for limiting the effect. J Pharmacol Exp Ther 179: 474–483
29. Holford NHG, Sheiner LB (1982) Kinetics of pharmacological response. Pharmac Ther 16: 143–166
30. Holley FO and van Steennis C (1988) Postoperative analgesia with fentanyl: pharmacokinetics and pharmacodynamics of constant rate i.v. and transdermal delivery. Br J Anaesth 60: 608–613
31. Hudson RJ (1986) Variability of fentanyl pharmacokinetics in neonates (letter). Anesth Analg 65: 1369–1370
32. Hudson RJ, Thomson IR, Cannon JG, Friesen RM, Meatherall RC (1986) Pharmacokinetics of fentanyl in patients undergoing abdominal aortic surgery. Anesthesiology 64: 334–338
33. Hug CC Jr (1985) Lipid solubility, pharmacokinetics, and the EEG: are you better off today than you were four years ago? Anesthesiology 62: 221–226
34. Hug CC Jr, Murphy MR (1981) Tissue redistribution of fentanyl and its termination of effects in rats. Anesthesiology 55: 369–375
35. Hull C (1983) The pharmacokinetics of alfentanil in man. Br J Anaesth 55: 157–164
36. Hynynen M (1987) Binding of fentanyl and alfentanil to the extracorporeal circuit. Acta Anaesthesiol Scand 31: 706–710
37. Hynynen M, Takkunen O, Salmenpera M, Haataja H, Heinonen J (1986) Continuous infusion of fentanyl or alfentanil for coronary artery surgery. Plasma opiate concentrations, haemodynamics and postoperative course. Br J Anaesth 58: 1252–1259
38. Johnson KL, Ericson JP, Holley FO, Scott JC (1984) Fentanyl pharmacokinetics in the pediatric population. Anesthesiology 61: A441
39. Justins DM, Knott C, Luthman J, Reynolds F (1983) Epidural versus intramuscular fentanyl: analgesia and pharmacokinetics in labour. Anaesthesia 38: 937–942
40. Koehntop DE, Rodman JH, Brundage DM, Hegland MG, Buckley JJ (1986) Pharmacokinetics of fentanyl in neonates. Anesth Analg 65: 227–232
41. Koren G, Crean P, Klein J, Goresky G, Villamater J, MacLeod SM (1984) Sequestration of fentanyl by the cardiopulmonary bypass. Eur J Clin Pharmacol 27: 27–51
42. Kowalski SR, Gourlay GK (1990) The stability of fentanyl in glass and plastic containers and with the components of a patient controlled analgesia pump. Am J Hosp Pharm 47: 1584–1587
43. Kowalski SR, Gourlay GK, Cherry DA, McLean CF (1987) A rapid gas liquid chromatographic method for the determination of fentanyl concentration suitable for use in studies involving acute and chronic pain. J Pharmacol Methods 18: 347–355
44. Kumar K, Morgan DJ, Crankshaw DP (1987) Determination of fentanyl and alfentanil in plasma by high performance liquid chromatography with ultraviolet detection. J Chromatogr 419: 464–468
45. Lampl E, Garen C, Levron P, Pathier D, Cousin MT (1986) Pharmacokinetics du fentanyl administre par voie peridurale chez la femme en travail. J Gynecol Obstet Biol Reprod Paris 15: 603–607
46. Latasch L, Luders S (1989) Transdermal fentanyl against postoperative pain. Acta Anaesthesiol Belg 40: 113–119
47. Lehmann KA (1984) Fentanyl: Kinetik und Dynamik. Perimed, Erlangen

48. Lehmann KA (1985) Opioid-Plasmakonzentrationen und pharmakodynamische Wirkung. Fortschr Med 103: 938–942
49. Lehmann KA, Hunger L, Brandt K, Daub D (1983) Biotransformation of fentanyl. III. Influence of chronic drug administration upon distribution, metabolism and excretion in the rat. Anaesthesist 32: 165–173
50. Lehmann KA, Moseler G, Daub D (1981) Biotransformation of fentanyl. I. Metabolism by mouse tissue homogenates In Vitro. Anaesthesist 30: 461–466
51. Lehmann KA, Schmitz KF, Daub D (1983) The disposition of fentanyl in human blood. Anaesthesist 32: 329–334
52. Lehmann KA, Weski C, Hunger L, Heinrich C, Daub D (1982) Biotransformation of fentanyl. II. Acute drug interactions in rats and men. Anaesthesist 31: 221–227
53. Lehmann KA, Heinrich C, van Heiss R (1988) Balanced anesthesia and patient controlled postoperative analgesia with fentanyl: minimum effective concentrations, accumulation and acute tolerance. Acta Anaesthesiol Belg 39: 11–23
54. Maitre PO, Stanski DR (1988) Bayesian forecasting improves the prediction of intraoperative plasma concentrations of fentanyl. Anesthesiology 69: 652–658
55. Maitre PO, Vozeh S, Heykants J, Stanski DR (1987) Population kinetics of alfentanil: the average dose plasma concentration relationship and interindividual variability in patients. Anesthesiology 66: 3–12
56. Mather LE, Runciman WB (1985) The physiological basis of pharmacokinetics: Concepts and tools. In: Stoeckel HO (ed) Quantitation, modelling and control in anaesthesia. Georg Thieme, Stuttgart, pp 12–40
57. Mather LE, Selby DG, Runciman WB (1990) The effects of propofol and of thiopentone anaesthesia on the regional kinetics of pethidine in the sheep. Br J Anaesth 66: 365–372
58. Mather LE (1983) Clinical pharmacokinetics of fentanyl and its newer derivatives. Clin Pharmacokinet 8: 422–446
59. McClain DA, Hug CC Jr (1980) Intravenous fentanyl kinetics. Clin Pharmacol Ther 28: 206–114
60. Meuldermans WEG, Hurkmans RMA, Heykants JJP (1982) Plasma protein binding and distribution of fentanyl, sufentanil, alfentanil and lofentanil in blood. Arch Int Pharm Ther 257: 4–19
61. Meyer-Breiting P, Leuwer M (1990) Fentanyl-Gabe zur Narkoseeinleitung bei Sectio caesarea. Pharmakokinetik und Pharmakodynamik bei Mutter und Kind. Anaesthesist 39: 144–150
62. Miser AW, Narang PK, Dothage JA, Young RC, Sindelar W, Miser JS (1989) Transdermal fentanyl for pain control in patients with cancer Pain 37: 15–21
63. Nishitateno K, Ngai SH, Finck AD, Berkowitz BA (1979) Pharmacokinetics of morphine: concentrations in the serum and the brain of the dog during hyperventilation. Anesthesiology 50: 520–523
64. Plezia PM, Kramer TH, Linford J, Hameroff SR (1989) Transdermal fentanyl: pharmacokinetics and preliminary clinical evaluation. Pharmacotherapy 9: 2–9
65. Raemer DB, Buschman A, Varvel JR, Philip BK, Johnson MD, Stein DA, Shafer SL (1990) The prospective use of population pharmacokinetics in a computer-driven infusion system for alfentanil. 73: 66–72
66. Reilly CS, Wood AJ, Wood M (1985) Variability of fentanyl pharmacokinetics in man. Computer predicted plasma concentrations for three intravenous dosage regimens. Anaesthesia 40: 837–843
67. Roerig DL, Kotrly KJ, Ahlf SB, Dawson CA, Kampine JP (1989) Effect of propranolol on the first pass uptake of fentanyl in the human and rat lung. Anesthesiology 71: 62–68
68. Roerig DL, Kotrly KJ, Vucins EJ, Ahlf SB, Dawson CA, Kampine JP (1987) First pass uptake of fentanyl, meperidine and morphine in the human lung. Anesthesiology 67: 466–472

69. Runcimann WB, Mather LE, Ilsley AH, Carapetis R, McLean CF (1984) A sheep preparation for studying the interaction of regional blood flow and drug disposition. II: Experimental applications. Br J Anaesth 56: 1117–1129
70. Runciman WB, Mather LE (1987) Effects of anaesthesia and drug disposition. In: Feldman SA, Scurr CF, Paton W (eds) Mechanism of action of drugs in anaesthetic practice. Edward Arnold, London, pp 87–122
71. Schmitt H, Batz G, Knoll R, Danner U, Brandt M (1990) Plasma level changes of fentanyl and midazolam after release of a prolonged thigh torniquet. Acta Anaesth Scand 34: 104–108
72. Schneider E, Brune K (1985) Distribution of fentanyl in rats: an autoradiographic study. Naunyn-Schmiedebergs Arch Pharmacol 331: 359–363
73. Schüttler J (1981) Klinische Pharmacokinetik von Fentanyl unter besonderer Berücksichtigung eines respiratorischen Rebound-Phänomens. Thesis: Rheinische Friedrich-Wilhelms-Universität, Bonn
74. Schüttler J, White PF (1984) Optimization of the radioimmunoassays for measuring fentanyl and alfentanil in human serum. Anesthesiology 61: 315–320
75. Schwilden H, Stoeckel H (1985) The derivation of EEG parameters for modelling and control of anaesthetic drug effect. In: Stoeckel HO (ed) Quantitation, modelling and control in anaesthesia. Georg Thieme, Stuttgart, pp 160–169
76. Scott JC, Ponganis KV, Stanski DR (1985) EEG quantitation of narcotic effect: The comparative pharmacodynamics of fentanyl and alfentanil. Anesthesiology 62: 234–241
77. Scott JC, Stanski DR (1987) Decreased fentanyl and alfentanil dose requirements with age. A simultaneous pharmacokinetic and pharmacodynamic evaluation. J Pharmacol Exp Ther 240: 159–166
78. Sebel PS (1981) Fentanyl anaesthesia in cardiac surgery. MD Thesis: University of Amsterdam
79. Singh AK, Ashraf M, Granley K, Mishra U, Rao MM, Gordon B (1989) Screening and confirmation of drugs in horse urine by using a simple column extraction procedure. J Chromatogr 473: 215–226
80. Singleton MA, Rosen JI, Fischer DM (1984) Pharmacokinetics of fentanyl for infants and adults. Anesthesiology 61: A440
81. Singleton MA, Rosen JI, Fischer DM (1988) Pharmacokinetics of fentanyl in the elderly. Br J Anaesth 60: 619–622
82. Stanley TH, Hague B, Mock DL, Streisand JB, Bubbers S (1989) Oral transmucosal fentanyl citrate (lollipop) premedication in human volunteers. Anesth Analg 69: 21–27
83. Stanley TH, Leiman BC, Rawal N, Marcus MA, van den Nieuwenhuyzen M, Walford A, Cronau LH, Pace NL (1989) The effects of oral transmucosal fentanyl citrate premedication on preoperative behavioral responses and gastric volume and acidity in children. Anesth Analg 328–335
84. Taeger K, Weninger E, Schmelzer F, Adt M, Franke M, Peter K (1988) Pulmonary kinetics of fentanyl and alfentanil in surgical patients. Br J Anaesth 61: 425–434
85. Tozer TN (1981) Concepts basic to pharmacokinetics. Pharmac Ther 12: 109–131
86. Tucker GT, Mather LE (1988) Properties, absorption and disposition of local anesthetics. In: Cousins MJ, Bridenbaugh PO (eds) Neural blockade, 2nd edition. Lippincott, Philadelphia, pp 47–110
87. Upton M, Mather LE, Runciman WB (1987) The influence of drug sorption on pharmacokinetic studies of chlormethiazole and lignocaine. J Pharm Pharmacol 39: 485–487
88. Upton RN, Mather LE, Runciman WB, Nancarrow C, Carapetis RJ (1988) The use of mass balance principles to describe regional drug distribution and elimination. J Pharmacokin Biopharm 16: 13–29
89. Upton RN, Runciman WB, Mather LE (1987) A relationship between some physicochemical properties of ionisable drugs and their sorption into medical plastics. Aust J Hosp Pharm 17: 267–272

90. Varvel JR, Shafer SL, Hwang SS, Coen PA, Stanski DR (1989) Absorption characteristics of transdermally administered fentanyl. Anesthesiology 70: 928–934
91. Vella LM, Knott C, Reynolds F (1986) Transfer of fentanyl across the rabbit placenta. Effect of umbilical flow and concurrent drug administration. Br J Anaesth 58: 49–54
92. von Bormann B, Ratthey K, Schwetlick G, Schneider C, Müller W (1988) Postoperative pain therapy by transdermal fentanyl. Anasth Intensivther Notfallmed 23: 3–8
93. Wagner JG (1981) History of pharmacokinetics. Pharmac Ther 12: 537–562
94. Weinberg DS, Inturrisi CE, Reidenberg B, Moulin DE, Nip TJ (1988) Sublingual absorption of selected opioid analgesics. Clin Pharmacol Ther 44: 335–342
95. Woestenborghs RJH, Stanski DR, Scott JC, Heykants JJP (1987) Assay methods for fentanyl in serum: gas liquid chromatography versus radioimmunoassay. Anesthesiology 67: 85–90
96. Woods WE, Tai HH, Tai C, Weckman T, Wood T, Barios H, Blake JW, Tobin T (1986) High sensitivity radioimmunoassay screening method for fentanyl. Am J Vet Res 47: 2180–2183
97. Worsley MH, Macleod AD, Brodie MJ, Asbury AJ, Clark C (1990) Inhaled fentanyl as a method of analgesia. Anaesthesia 45: 449–451

Premedication and Pain Management with Oral Transmucosal Fentanyl

J. B. STREISAND

Introduction

Until recently, the treatment of moderate to severe pain had been limited to intramuscular or intravenous bolus administration of narcotic analgesics. However, a greater understanding of the pharmacokinetics and dynamics of narcotic analgesics combined with prolific biomedical technological research have resulted in the development of several devices that administer opioids noninvasively. Compared to traditional parenteral techniques, these new opioid delivery systems have several advantages: improved patient convenience and compliance, minimal discomfort on delivery, better bioavailability, heightened safety, fewer peaks and valleys in drug plasma levels and therefore more effective drug action.

One such delivery device, Oral Transmucosal Fentanyl Citrate (OTFC), utilizes oral mucosa as a site for drug delivery. OTFC units consist of a lozenge with a handle and are of uniform size and shape. They are manufactured by dissolving fentanyl citrate crystals into a sucrose-based solution. After mixing to ensure uniform distribution of the drug, the mixture is poured into molds, a handle added, and the units allowed to cool and harden. As a patient consumes OTFC, fentanyl is released to the oral mucosa and absorbed directly into the systemic circulation. The remaining fentanyl is swallowed and dispatched to the stomach and gut where it is absorbed and undergoes first-pass hepatic metabolism.

OTFC has been undergoing clinical trials in the United States since 1985. It is expected that clinical trials will start in Europe in the near future. Although first developed for pediatric premedication, other clinical applications for the device have emerged. These include analgesia for acute postoperative and breakthrough cancer pain, and sedation and analgesia for emergency room and other painful diagnostic and therapeutic procedures not requiring a general anesthetic. This chapter reviews and summarizes data from volunteer and clinical studies using OTFC.

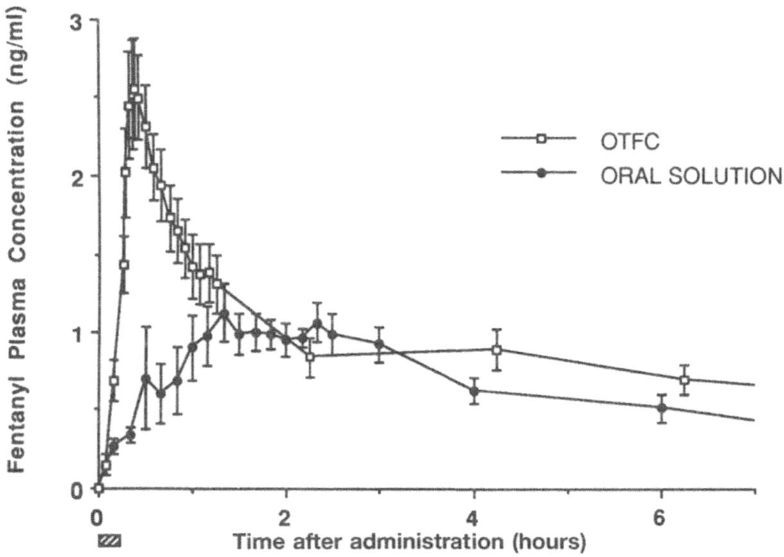

Fig. 1. Mean and SEM of plasma fentanyl concentrations following OTFC, 15 μg/kg. The crosshatched bar represents consumption time of OTFC. For comparison, plasma fentanyl concentrations following a swallowed fentanyl solution, 15 μg/kg, are also shown

Pharmacokinetics of OTFC

To understand the safe and effective use of new drug delivery devices such as OTFC, it is necessary to understand their biopharmaceutics in order to guide the selection of dosages. Streisand et al. determined fentanyl plasma concentrations, absorption and bioavailability of OTFC (15 μg/kg) in human volunteers [14]. Fentanyl plasma concentrations rapidly increase to 2.8 ± 1.0 ng/ml 23 min after administration, then decrease to less than 1 ng/ml approximately 1 h later (Fig. 1, Table 1). A plasma concentration of 1 ng/ml, which generally results in postsurgical analgesia [9] is attained *during* OTFC consumption. Oral mucosal absorption explains the rapid uptake of fentanyl from OTFC into the systemic circulation (Fig. 2). Fentanyl that is swallowed and absorbed in the gastrointestinal tract undergoes hepatic first-pass metabolism. This explains why the bioavailability of OTFC is significantly greater than the bioavailability of swallowed fentanyl (Table 1).

Table 1. Bioavailability and peak plasma fentanyl concentrations (mean ± SD) following OTFC and oral solution administrations

	OTFC	Oral solution
C_{max} (ng/ml)	2.8 ± 1.0	1.6 ± 0.6
T_{max} (min)	23 ± 3	101 ± 49
Bioavailability	0.50 ± 0.1	0.32 ± 0.1

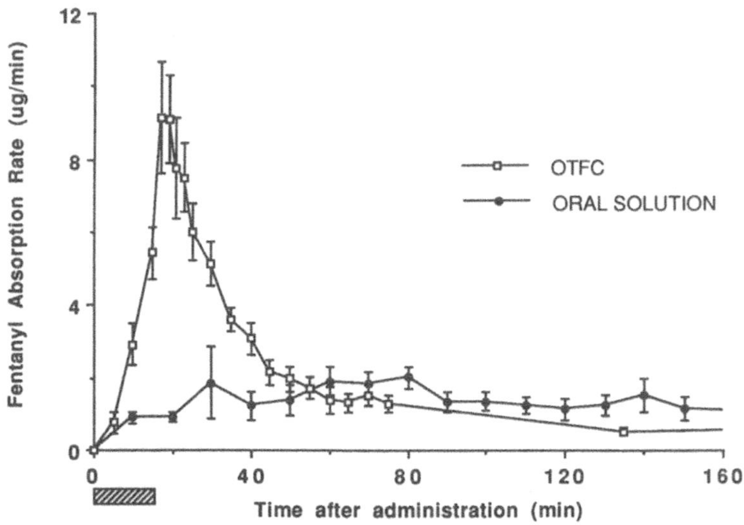

Fig. 2. Mean and SEM of fentanyl absorption rate following OTFC, 15 μg/kg. The crosshatched bar represents consumption time of OTFC. For comparison, absorption rate following a swallowed fentanyl solution, 15 μg/kg, is also shown

Table 2. Terminal elimination half-lives (mean ± SD) after four routes of fentanyl administration

Route	Half-life (h)
Intravenous	7.1 ± 1.7
OTFC	7.7 ± 5.2
Oral	7.8 ± 2.1
Transdermal	16.6 ± 3.7

There is no difference in the elimination of fentanyl after OTFC or iv administration (Table 2). Thus fentanyl is not sequestered in the oral mucosa after OTFC administration. On the other hand, transdermal fentanyl leaves a fentanyl "depot" in the skin, accounting for its long elimination half-life [19].

Absorption of fentanyl from OTFC through oral mucosal membranes is complex and involves numerous factors. During OTFC consumption, rate of sucking and saliva production (which is affected by taste and pH of the OTFC matrix) influence dissolution of the matrix. Fentanyl in saliva is then exposed to the absorptive surfaces of the mouth including buccal, sublingual, gingival and tongue mucosae. Although not specifically characterized for fentanyl, drug permeability is generally highest in the buccal and sublingual areas and lowest at the gingiva and tongue [8]. The remaining unabsorbed fentanyl is then swallowed. How much saliva is immediately swallowed without adequate exposure to the mucosal surfaces is a critical factor in the overall absorption process and probably explains much of the interpatient variability in fentanyl absorption from OTFC. In general, diffusion through biologic membranes occurs most favorably when a drug is in its nonionized, most lipid-soluble form. Ionization of fentanyl (a weak base with a pKa of 8.4) is dependent upon environmental pH. Higher pH favors the unionized form of fentanyl and enhances mucosal penetration. The pH in the mouth after OTFC administration results from a combination of saliva, whose pH varies from 6.5 to 6.9 [4], and the dissolved sucrose base, whose pH ranges from 5.5 to 6. Finally, changes in blood- and lymph flow to sites of absorption will also influence the transport of fentanyl into the systemic circulation.

Clinical Experience

Initial Volunteer Studies

The first human evaluations with OTFC were done in 28 human volunteers in an open-label, nonrandomized study [17]. Volunteers consumed OTFC doses of 0.5, 1.0, 2.0, 4.0, or 5.0 mg. Dose-related analgesia (determined by a graded electrical stimulus) and respiratory depression occurred concurrent with the appearance of significant fentanyl concentrations in the blood (range 0.8–23 ng/ml). No circulatory changes or muscular rigidity transpired. All doses produced nasal pruritus, but nausea and vomiting was seen only in the 2, 4, and 5 mg doses. These higher doses were also associated with occasional apnea and oxygen desaturation. However, doses of 0.5 and 1.0 mg (5–15 μg/kg) yielded significant analgesia and sedation for 1–2 h with little respiratory depression. Results from this initial study indicated further clinical investigation with the lower OTFC dose ranges (5–15 μg/kg) was warranted.

Pediatric Premedication

Since this noninvasive delivery system has obvious appeal in children, surgical premedication was the first clinical application of OTFC that was investigated. Inasmuch as this was to be the first clinical exposure of OTFC in children, an open-label, nonrandomized study was undertaken to determine the appropriate OTFC dose for pediatric premedication [15]. Forty-four children scheduled to undergo ENT, ophthalmologic, urologic, or orthopedic surgery were administered OTFC in dose ranges of 5–10, 10–15, 15–20, and 20–25 μg/kg 30–90 min prior to operation. Activity (sedation) and anxiety scores, vital signs, and oxygen saturation were measured at baseline and at 15-min intervals until the patients were taken to the operating room. OTFC was readily accepted and provided dose-related reductions in preoperative activity with significance 30 min after administration (Fig. 3). Vital signs remained unchanged during the preoperative evaluation period except in the

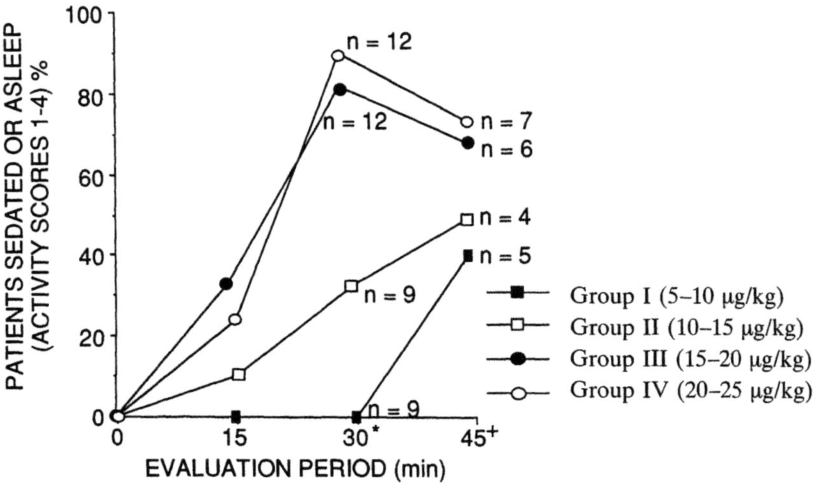

Fig. 3. Percentage of patients sedated or asleep as a function of time in children premedicated with oral transmucosal fentanyl citrate (OTFC) in the doses indicated. $*P = 0.0001$, $+ P = 0.0002$, when all patients considered as one group as compared to baseline, Wilcoxon test

highest dose range administered (20–25 μg/kg) where oxygen saturation and respiratory rate were significantly reduced from baseline and occasional oxygen desaturation (<90 %) occurred (3 of 12 patients). OTFC caused dose-independent preoperative pruritus in over 90 % of patients and postoperative pruritus (33 %–70 %), nausea (30 %–58 %), and vomiting (50 %–80 %). The results from this study suggested that 15–20 μg/kg was the optimal dose range of OTFC in healthy children for optimizing onset (18 min) and magnitude (92 % calm, sedated, or asleep) of preoperative sedation and minimizing preoperative respiratory side effects (lowest respiratory rate = 16 breaths/min and lowest oxygen saturation 95 %).

In total, OTFC has been administered to children for premedication over 800 times in 13 clinical trials at nine hospitals in the United States. Healthy children and those with congenital heart disease have participated in a variety of blinded, well-controlled clinical studies (in both inpatient and outpatient settings) comparing OTFC to placebo and other popular premedication oral cocktails [12, 15, 18, 5, 2, 7]. In summary, OTFC doses of 10–20 μg/kg produced significant decreases in activity (sedation) and apprehension 20–40 min after administration when compared to placebo and was equally or more effective than other premedication regimens [12, 18, 5, 3, 7]. Although statistically significant decreases in respiratory rate and oxygen saturation were reported in some studies, these were small and of little clinical consequence [18, 5, 2]. OTFC helped facilitate a smooth, calm transition from the preoperative holding area through induction of anesthesia [5, 7]. In most studies, recovery times were not different following administration of OTFC, placebo or other premedications [12, 15, 5, 2]. However, discharge from an outpatient center was slightly prolonged by OTFC administration (299 min OTFC vs 197 min placebo) because children who received placebo were able to tolerate fluids sooner postoperatively than the children who received OTFC [2]. Analgesic requirements in the postanesthesia recovery room were markedly reduced by OTFC premedication [12, 15, 18, 5, 2]. Pruritus, nausea, and vomiting were the most common side effects reported. Pruritus was usually limited to the nose and face, occurred preoperatively (60%–90% incidence), and coincided with the onset of sedation, but was rarely found in the postanesthesia recovery room [12, 15, 18, 5, 2]. While preoperative emesis rarely occurred (5%–15% incidence [2, 6]), postoperative emesis was reported as high as 64% [7]. Interestingly, in one study, emptying the stomach by intraoperative orogastric suction markedly reduced the incidence of postoperative emesis to 6% [18].

Does administration of OTFC for premedication increase the risk of aspiration during the perioperative period? This important concern was addressed by Stanley et al. [18]. Following premedication with OTFC, a placebo unit, or nothing, for premedication, the authors determined gastric pH and volume by orogastric suction immediately after tracheal intubation. Gastric pH was similar in all three groups. Despite a higher gastric volume found after OTFC and placebo units compared to no premedication (15 and 16 vs 8 ml, respectively), there was no difference between groups in the percentage of children considered "at risk" (pH <2.5 and gastric volume >0.4 ml/kg) for acid aspiration (Table 3). To date, in over 800 OTFC administrations during clinical trials, no occurrences of aspiration have been reported.

Table 3. Gastric volume and pH data in 53 children receiving premedication with oral transmucosal fentanyl citrate (OTFC), a placebo unit, or no premedication

	Group A (No premedication)	Group B (OTFC)	Group C (Placebo)
N	16	18	19
Gastric volume (ml/kg)	0.30	0.57*	0.54
Mean ± SD)	± 0.20	± 0.39	± 0.45
Patients with pH <2.5			
Number	12	13	18
Percent	75	72	95
Patients with pH >2.5			
Number	1	2	1
Percent	6	11	5
Dry cases, no pH measured			
Number	3	3	0
Percent	19	17	0
Safe cases*			
Number	4	5	1
Percent	25	28	5

* pH >2.5 and gastric volume <0.4 ml/kg

Cancer Pain

Poor control of pain due to malignant disease is a worldwide problem affecting up to 70% of patients with cancer, despite the use of commonly available analgesics [20]. One of the difficulties pursuant to the management of cancer pain is that few people are in a "steady state". Pain may increase episodically from changes in activity (incident pain) or without apparent reason (breakthrough pain). If efforts are made to provide analgesia for all circumstances by increasing time-contingent doses of long-acting analgesics, adverse side effects such as oversedation, nausea, or constipation can override any therapeutic gains. Presently available oral, rectal, or sublingual analgesic formulations have lengthy onset times and therefore are unable to provide rapid boosts in analgesia appropriate to a patient's specific circumstance. OTFC is a rapidly-absorbed, relatively-short-acting, easily-administered and potent, yet titratable, analgesic delivery system. These properties of OTFC suggest that it would be a valuable adjunct for the management of breakthrough and incident cancer pain.

To study this indication for OTFC, ten patients with advanced cancer and breakthrough or incident pain received OTFC, 10–15 μg/kg, on four of five different occasions over 2 days in an open-label study [6]. Significant reduction in pain scores as measured by a pain descriptive scale, the McGill-Melzack scale, and a numeric visual analogue scale were seen at all evaluations from 5 to 120 min following administration. In addition, onset of analgesia was rapid, within 10 min of administration, and there were no requests for rescue analgesics. The incidence of respiratory and other opioid side effects was minimal, perhaps because of the tolerance to opioids often developed by this patient population. The results from this study and from a pilot case study [1] warrant the further clinical investigation of OTFC for cancer pain management.

Children undergoing repeated lumbar punctures (LP) and bone-marrow aspirations (BSA) as a necessary part of the diagnosis and treatment of childhood cancer often declare that the anxiety and discomfort associated with these procedures are worse than the disease itself [13]. Despite this problem, there has been no uniform approach to the provision of sedation and analgesia for children undergoing painful procedures. Previous experience with OTFC for surgical premedication in children suggested its use in this arena. Schechter et al. administered OTFC, 12.5 μg/kg, to children prior to LP or BSA in an open-label pilot study [13]. Average pain scores (maximum 10) were reduced from 8.2 (in a prior similar procedure without premedication) to 3.9 by OTFC administration. These encouraging results have led the same investigators to proceed with a placebo-controlled, double-blinded study with OTFC for sedation and analgesia prior to painful procedures in children with cancer.

New Developments

Recently completed pilot studies suggest OTFC may be helpful in providing analgesia for emergency room procedures [11] and acute postoperative pain [10]. Further studies in these areas are being planned. Ongoing pharmaceutical research is focusing on determining factors which enhance mucosal absorption of fentanyl. Initial results suggest that a change in pH or the use of permeation enhancers in the matrix formulation may speed the absorption of fentanyl from an OTFC matrix (J. Zhang, Anesta Corp., personal communication). Ideally, as adaptations are made in the formulation of OTFC, increased control over the rate of appearance of fentanyl in the blood will improve "tailoring" of this drug-delivery system to specific clinical situations. Clearly, the oral mucosa is an underutilized site for drug administration. In the future, one can expect the development of other new drug formulations for transmucosal drug delivery.

References

1. Ashburn MA, Fine PG, Stanley TH (1989) Oral transmucosal fentanyl citrate for the treatment of breakthrough cancer pain: A case report. Anesthesiology 71: 615–617
2. Ashburn MA, Olson L, Fine PG, Stanley TH (1990) The clinical evaluation of the compassionate use of oral transmucosal fentanyl citrate (OTFC) for the treatment of breakthrough cancer pain. Pain 5 (Suppl): S353
3. Ashburn MA, Streisand JB, Tarver S, Mears S, Mulder S, Wilms-Floet A, Elwyn RA, Pace NL, Stanley TH (In Press) Oral transmucosal fentanyl citrate for premedication in pediatric outpatients. Can J Anesth
4. Birkhed D, Heintze U (1989) Human Saliva. In: Tenovuo JO (ed) Clinical chemistry and microbiology. CRC Press Inc., Florida, p 53
5. Feld LH, Champeau MW, van Steennis CA, Scott JC (1989) Preanesthetic medication in children: A comparison of oral transmucosal fentanyl citrate versus placebo. Anesthesiology 71: 374–377
6. Fine PG, Marcus M, DeBoer AJ, Van Der Oord B (In Press) An open label study of oral transmucosal fentanyl citrate (OTFC) for the treatment of breakthrough cancer pain. Pain
7. Friesen RH, Lockhart CH (eds) Clinical trial of oral transmucosal fentanyl citrate for premedication of pediatric day surgery patients. Droperidol for control of nausea. Section on Anesthesiology, Program for scientific sessions, American Academy of Pediatrics, 27–29 April 1990, Seattle
8. Gibaldi M, Kanig J (1965) Absorption of drugs through the oral mucosa. J Oral Therap Pharmacol 1 (4): 440–450
9. Gourlay GK, Kowalski SR, Plummer JL, Cousins MJ, Armstrong PJ (1988) Fentanyl blood concentration-analgesic response relationship in the treatment of postoperative pain. Anesth Analg 67: 329–378
10. Lind GH, Ashburn MA, Gillie MH, de Boer AJF, Stanley TH (In Press) Oral transmucosal fentanyl citrate (OTFC) for the treatment of postoperative pain. Anesthesiology
11. Lind GH, Marcus MA, Ashburn MA, Mears SL, Petersen B, Stanley TH (1990) Oral transmucosal fentanyl citrate for analgesia and anxiolysis in the emergency room. Anesth Analg 72: S241
12. Nelson PS, Streisand JB, Mulder SM, Pace NL, Stanley TH (1989) Comparison of oral transmucosal fentanyl citrate and an oral solution of meperidine, diazepam and atropine for premedication in children. Anesthesiology 70: 616–621

13. Schechter NL, Weisman SJ, Rosenblum M, Beck A, Altman A, Quinn J, Conrad PF (1990) Sedation for painful procedures in children with cancer using the fentanyl lollipop: A preliminary report. In: Tyler DC, Krane EJ (eds) Advances in pain research therapy, Vol 15, Raven Press, New York
14. Streisand JB, Ashburn MA, LeMaire L, Varvel JR, Stanley TH, Tarver S (1989) Bioavailability and absorption of oral transmucosal fentanyl citrate. Anesthesiology 71: A229
15. Streisand JB, Stanley TH, Hague B, van Vreeskwijk H, Ho GH, Pace NL (1989) Oral transmucosal fentanyl citrate premedication in children. Anesth Analg 69: 28–34
16. Streisand JB, Tarver SD, Varvel J, Demmink M, Hague BL (In Press) Oral transmucosal fentanyl citrate: Oral transmucosal vs gastrointestinal absorption. Anesthesiology
17. Stanley TH, Hague B, Mock DL, Streisand JB, Bubbers S, Dzelzkalns RR, Bailey PL, Pace NL, East KA, Ashburn MA (1989) Oral transmucosal fentanyl citrate (lollipop) premedication in human volunteers. Anesth Analg 69: 21–27
18. Stanley TH, Leiman BC, Rawal N, Marcus M, van den Neuwenhuyzen M, Walford A, Cronau L, Pace NL (1989) The effects of oral transmucosal fentanyl citrate premedication on preoperative behavioral responses and gastric volume and acidity in children. Anesth Analg 69: 328–335
19. Varvel JR, Shafer SL, Hwang SS, Coen PA, Stanski DR (1989) Absorption characteristics of transdermally administered fentanyl. Anesthesiology 70: 928–934
20. Ventafridda V, Tamburine M, Caraceni A, De Conno F, Naldi F (1987) A validation study of the WHO method for cancer pain relief. Cancer 59: 850–856

Transdermal Fentanyl: an Overview of Pharmacokinetics, Efficacy and Safety

M. Southam, S. Gupta, M. Knowles, and S. S. Hwang

Introduction

The development of Transdermal Therapeutic System (Fentanyl) (TTS fentanyl) has combined fentanyl, an opioid that has been used for over 20 years, with a transdermal drug delivery system [Alza Corporation, Palo Alto, CA]. The system controls release of fentanyl to maintain a continuous and steady supply of drug through the skin. Application of a new TTS fentanyl every 72 h can provide the sustained and relatively constant serum fentanyl concentrations associated with continuous intravenous or subcutaneous opioid delivery but without invasive procedures or special equipment.

The United States Food and Drug Administration has recently approved TTS fentanyl for the management of chronic pain in patients requiring opioid analgesics. Including TTS fentanyl in the armamentarium of drugs and routes of administration for opioid analgesia is a significant advance, particularly for patients with pain-producing malignancies, e.g., primary bone tumors, and indeed for most cancer patients who experience significant pain late in the course of their disease. These patients often require a change of drugs to take advantage of incomplete cross-tolerance among drugs and generally at least two routes of analgesic administration [3].

This chapter provides an integrated overview of the pharmacokinetics, efficacy, and safety of TTS fentanyl.

Pharmacokinetics

The single- and multiple-dose pharmacokinetics of TTS fentanyl were evaluated in postsurgical and cancer patients. When the TTS is applied, the skin under it absorbs fentanyl, which initially concentrates in upper skin layers. The drug then becomes available to the systemic circulation and serum concentrations increase gradually. Following the first application, fentanyl can be detected in serum (0.2 ng/ml) after 1–2 h, and fentanyl concentrations generally plateau between 12 and 24 h after transdermal application [18, 15]. The concentrations achieved are proportional (approximately 0.5, 1, 1.5 and 2 ng/ml for the 25, 50, 75, and 100 μ/h systems respectively) [Alza Corporation data]. These relatively steady concentrations are maintained for the 72 h application period [8].

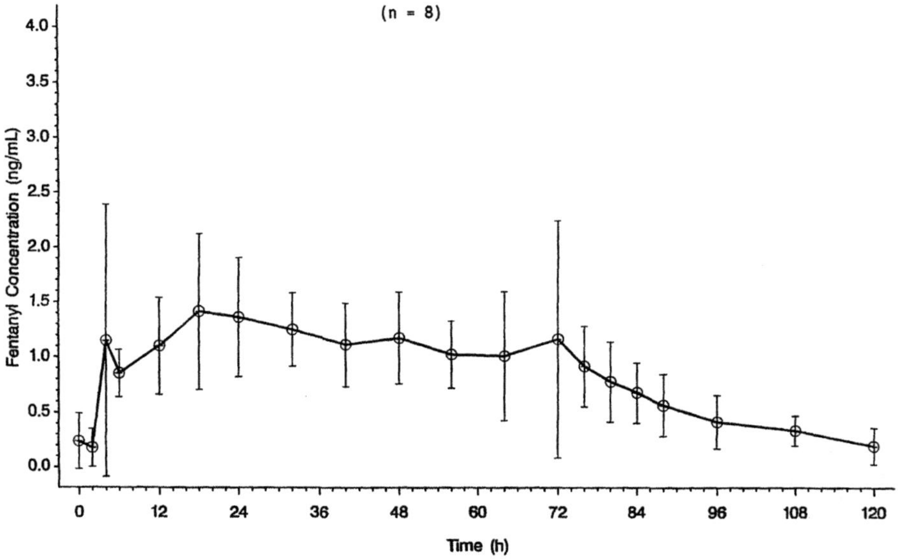

Fig. 1. Mean (SD) serum fentanyl concentration for one TTS fentanyl, 75 µg/h, applied for 3 days

Serum concentrations reach steady state by the second dose, and these concentrations are maintained with repeated application [Alza Corporation data]. The kinetics remain unchanged over time.

Following system removal, serum fentanyl concentrations decline gradually, falling about 50 % in approximately 17 h [18]. Because fentanyl continues

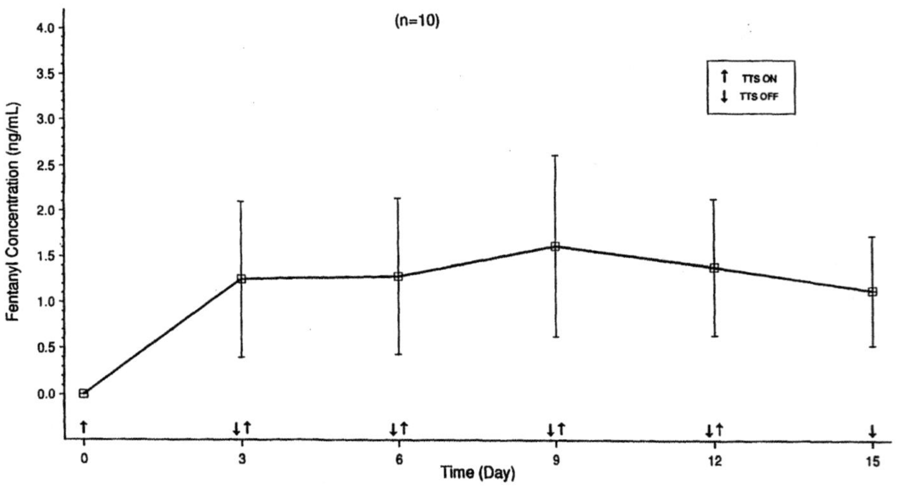

Fig. 2. Mean observed serum fentanyl concentrations during five consecutive 3 day TTS fentanyl 100 µg/h applications

to be absorbed from the skin, it disappears more slowly from the serum after transdermal administration than after an intravenous administration (apparent half-life is approximately 7 h) [18].

Fentanyl delivered transdermally is not metabolized by the skin and is 92 % bioavailable [18]; absorption continues throughout the entire 72 h dosing interval [18]. Serum fentanyl kinetics are linear within the dose range studied and do not change with repeated applications [Alza Corporation data].

Clinical Efficacy

The analgesic efficacy of fentanyl administered intravenously is well-established [12, 7, 4, 11]. The efficacy trials for transdermal fentanyl were undertaken in patients with acute postoperative pain or chronic cancer pain.

Acute Postoperative Pain

The efficacy of TTS fentanyl has been evaluated in eight controlled clinical trials including over 450 postoperative patients. The TTS fentanyl dose – 50, 75, or 100 μg/h – was selected for each trial based upon the severity of pain anticipated for a given surgical procedure (e.g., hysterectomy patients received the 50 μg/h dose and thoracotomy patients received the 100 μg/h dose).

Methods

The studies used a similar design and methodology to compare TTS fentanyl with placebo. All were double blind, randomized, parallel-group trials in patients undergoing surgical procedures expected to produce moderate to severe pain. A TTS fentanyl (50, 75 or 100 μg/h) or a transdermal placebo system was applied to the patient's upper torso 0–2 h before surgery with regional or general anesthesia. In the postoperative anesthesia recovery (PAR) room, patients in both treatment groups were eligible to receive an intravenous opioid titrated to their analgesic needs. After leaving PAR, patients received their supplementary analgesic via intramuscular injection or a patient controlled analgesic (PCA) device, depending on the study protocol.

The primary outcome measured was the amount of supplementary analgesic used by each treatment group. Pain intensity evaluations were included to assess the level of analgesia. Because both the active and placebo groups could be titrated to analgesia with a supplementary analgesic, no differences between treatment groups in pain intensity were anticipated. Patients and medical observers provided global rating of pain control for the entire 24 h treatment period.

Results

Morphine Use. The efficacy of TTS fentanyl was established in seven of nine clinical trials; in these seven the TTS fentanyl group used significantly less supplementary analgesic ($p < 0.1$) than patients in the TTS placebo group [16, 2, 1, 9, 10, Alza Corporation data]. The TTS placebo group used 2–4 times more supplementary analgesic than patients in the TTS fentanyl group. In the other two studies the mean supplementary analgesic was also lower in the TTS fentanyl group than in the placebo group, although the differences were not statistically significant [15, Alza Corporation data].

Figure 3 illustrates supplementary analgesic use in one clinical trial evaluating TTS fentanyl (100 μg/h) in patients undergoing major surgery (e.g., thoractomy) [Alza Corporation data]. Efficacy was demonstrated beginning in the immediate postoperative period and continuing throughout the period of TTS fentanyl application ($p < 0.01$). TTS fentanyl was effective alone (67 % of patients (or with minimal supplementation (23 % of patients); the lowest supplementation occurred in the 12–24 h period after TTS fentanyl application when serum fentanyl concentrations were highest.

When TTS fentanyl was removed after 24 h application, its analgesic effects persisted for another 12 h. The analgesic use by the active treatment group was statistically significantly less in the first 6 h after TTS removal. For an additional 6 h these patients continued to use analgesics at a lower rate than the placebo group, although differences between groups were not statistically significant. The sustained analgesia after system removal may be partially explained by the slow decline of serum fentanyl concentrations that occur after TTS removal. The 24–36 h data in Fig. 3 are representative of the majority of trials.

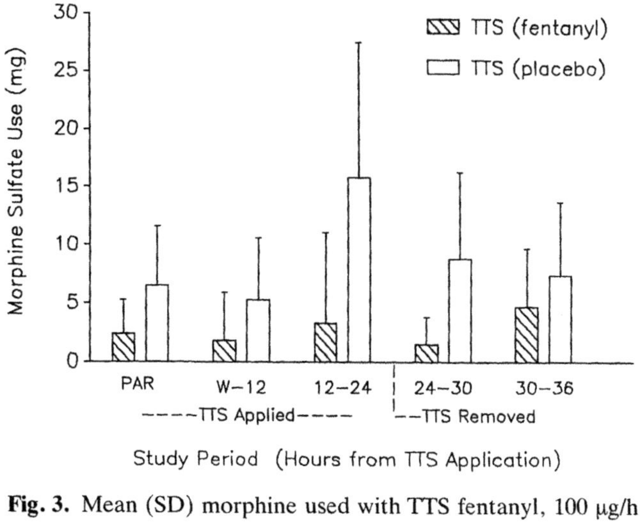

Fig. 3. Mean (SD) morphine used with TTS fentanyl, 100 μg/h, or placebo

Pain Intensity. Although placebo patients had more frequent access to supplemental analgesic than patients have in usual clinical practice, those using TTS fentanyl had significantly lower pain intensity ratings ($p < 0.01$) than the control group in all seven positive trials. In the four trials using a numeric scale (0–9), pain intensity ratings were 40 %–60 % lower for the TTS fentanyl group than for the placebo group. Patients using TTS fentanyl reported excellent pain control with mean pain intensity scores of 2–3 (scale 0–9) during the 12–24 h interval after TTS application.

Figure 4 illustrates pain intensity ratings from one clinical trial. In the 18–24 h period after TTS application, mean scores for patients receiving TTS fentanyl (100 μg/h) [Alza Corporation data] were 1.8 (SD = 1.8) versus 4.3 (SD = 2.1) for patients receiving TTS placebo ($p < 0.01$).

Global Pain Control Evaluation. In five of six clinical trials pain control was rated significantly better ($p < 0.05$) by patients using TTS fentanyl than by patients using a transdermal placebo plus an intramuscular or intravenous analgesic [Alza Corporation data]. Global pain control was evaluated as excellent or very good by more than twice as many patients in the active group as in the placebo group (60 %–88 % versus 22 %–38 %).

Serum Fentanyl Concentration-Effect Relationship. The relationship of serum fentanyl concentration to morphine use was evaluated in double blind trials. Statistically significant differences between the active and placebo groups in supplementary analgesic use were observed 0–2 h after surgery when mean serum fentanyl concentrations were in the minimum analgesic range (mean: 0.6 ng/ml) [6, Alza Corporation data]. These differences were maximal during the 12–14 h study when serum fentanyl concentrations plateaued.

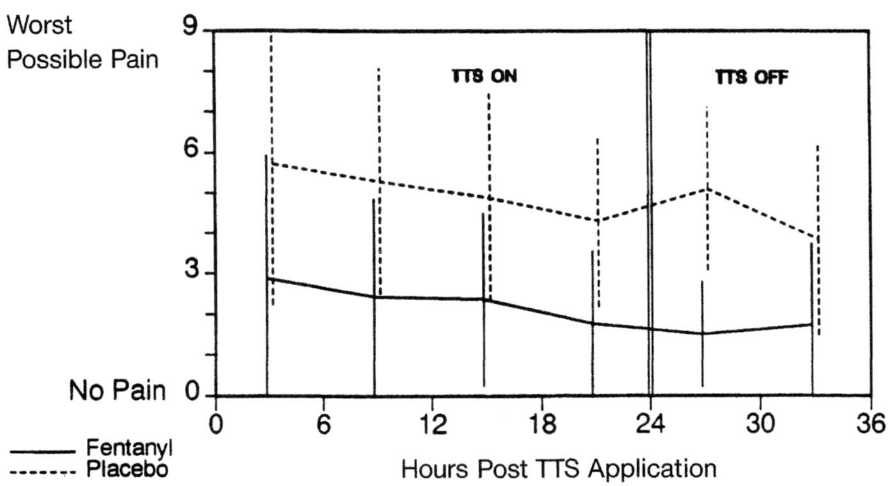

Fig. 4. Mean (SD) pain intensity ratings by patients with TTS Fentanyl, 100 μg/h, or placebo

Patients ($n = 206$) in five double blind trials were stratified on mean serum fentanyl concentration during a 12 h time interval. Patients with serum concentrations in the 0–0.75 ng/ml used an average of 11.7 mg morphine compared to an average of 8.3 mg for patients with serum concentrations over 1.75 ng/ml.

Chronic Cancer Pain

Methods

A multi-center, double-blind, cross-over trial was conducted to evaluate the efficacy of transdermally administered fentanyl for pain due to advanced cancer. Patients were hospitalized for cancer treatment. They were switched to a TTS fentanyl dose based upon an estimated analgesic equivalent of their previous daily analgesic intake and on their clinical presentation. For example, a patient who was on an oral morphine regimen of 180 mg/day was prescribed an initial TTS fentanyl dose of 50 μg/h. After stabilization on TTS fentanyl patients were randomized to a 1-week regimen of either TTS fentanyl or placebo and then crossed over to the alternative regimen for the following 1-week period. Supplementary analgesics were available during both phases of the study, and pain intensity was assessed.

Results

Thirty-five patients entered the trial; 23 completed the double-blind phase. There were no significant differences in morphine use between treatments; however, patients achieved significantly ($p < 0.04$) better pain control with TTS fentanyl plus rescue analgesics than with a placebo plus rescue analgesics. Four patients died, two patients required dose increase, and two patients on placebo dropped out due to inadequate pain control. An additional four patients were removed from the trial due to protocol violations [Alza Corporation data]. These data highlight some ethical and practical issues in placebo-controlled trials of two weeks' duration in patients with such severe disease that pain is likely to escalate and death is probable.

Experience in Clinical Practice with Cancer Patients

Supporting Evidence of Efficacy

A subsequent open-label multi-center trial in cancer patients was conducted using an A–B study design [13, 17]. Patients were titrated to acceptable analgesia with oral morphine. Those on other analgesia regimens (20 %) were converted to morphine using equivalency tables. The total daily morphine dose was used to convert patients to TTS fentanyl on the basis of an estimated morphine-to-fentanyl equivalency. They were then permitted morphine as needed. A patient who had not attained acceptable analgesia on morphine could be converted to a higher TTS fentanyl dose. The analgesic outcome was evaluated after 1 month of TTS fentanyl treatment by comparing the reduction of oral morphine use, pain intensity, and pain control satisfaction ratings with prestudy- and baseline values.

The results showed a statistically significant reduction ($p = 0.001$) in morphine use and in pain intensity scores 1 month after treatment initiation, compared to baseline. The mean pain intensity score 1 month after treatment initiation was 3.3 cm versus 4.6 cm at baseline ($p = 0.0194$). Pain intensity ratings were the same or better for 73 % of the patients (Fig. 5) who also reported good to excellent satisfaction with their pain control [Alza Corporation data].

Extent of Exposure

To date more than 17 000 patient days of TTS fentanyl have accrued in five clinical trials at ten different institutions. Patients have received TTS fentanyl doses in the range of 25 μg/h to 600 μg/h for 1 to 866 days. More than 50 % of these patients used TTS fentanyl for over 1 month and 10 % continued use for more than 1 year [Alza Corporation data].

Patients in these clinical trials were considered representative of many who will be candidates for treatment with TTS fentanyl. Though receiving opioids orally or parenterally, the majority were not achieving adequate control of

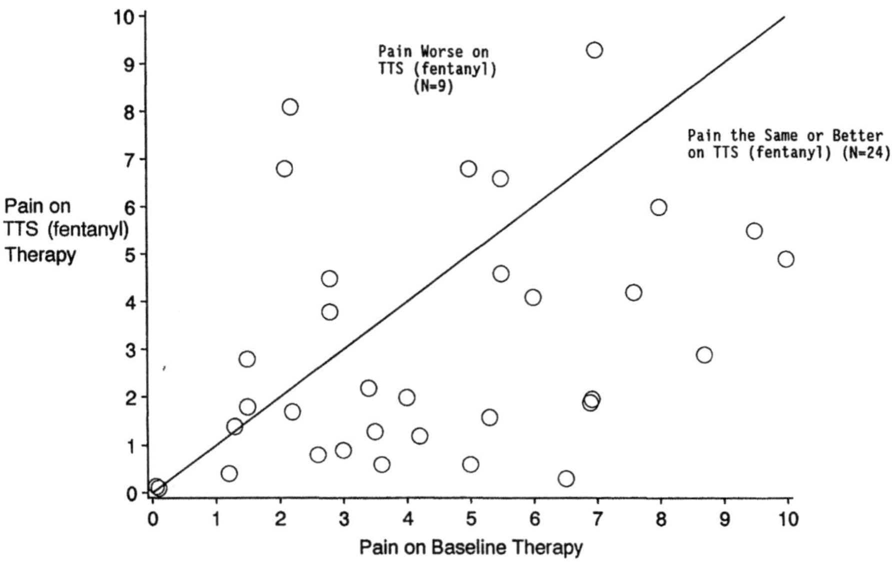

Fig. 5. Visual analogue pain scores: 1 month on TTS Fentanyl versus baseline

pain associated with cancer with conventional analgesic regimens and for this reason were considered for TTS fentanyl use.

More than half of the patients were 60 years of age or older (range: 16–81). The malignancies most frequently reported were those of the breast, lung, and gastrointestinal tract, and the prognosis of most patients was poor. All patients were receiving palliative therapy for cancer or associated symptoms.

Dose Selection

The initial TTS fentanyl dose was based upon each patient's clinical history, clinical presentation and previous analgesic requirement. The patient's total daily analgesic was calculated. If the analgesic was other than morphine, the dose was converted to an equivalent morphine dose using a standard equivalency table [5]. The daily morphine dose was then converted to a TTS fentanyl dose based on the scheme presented in Table 1. For example, patients whose daily oral morphine dose ranged from 315 to 404 mg, or whose parenteral dose ranged from 53 to 67 mg, were prescribed TTS fentanyl, 100 μg/h. Those whose pain was not well controlled with their previous analgesic could be prescribed a higher TTS fentanyl dose.

This method of conversion from conventional oral and parenteral opioids proved conservative and thus insured safety upon treatment initiation. No patient received an excessive initial dose which had to be decreased. In fact, approximately 50 % of patients required a dose titration upward after the first week of treatment [Alza Corporation data]. Since TTS fentanyl was available in 25 μg/h dose increments, patients could easily be individually titrated to an efficacious dose.

Table 1. TTS fentanyl dose prescription based upon daily morphine dose

Morphine oral, 24-h* (mg/day)	Morphine i.m., 24-h* (mg/day)	TTS fentanyl dose (μg/h)
45– 134	8– 22	25
135– 224	23– 37	50
225– 314	38– 52	75
315– 404	53– 67	100
405– 494	68– 82	125
495– 584	83– 97	150
585– 674	98–112	175
675– 764	113–127	200
765– 854	128–142	225
855– 944	143–157	250
945–1034	158–172	275
1035–1124	173–187	300

* A 10 mg i.m. or 60 mg oral dose of morphine every 4 h for 24 h (total 60 mg/day i.m. or 360 mg/day orally) was considered approximately equivalent to TTS fentanyl 100 μg/h

Safety

The safety of TTS fentanyl has been evaluated in 357 postoperative patients and 153 cancer patients for a total of 510 patients. Hypoventilation was the most serious adverse reaction, occurring in 13 (4 %) postoperative patients and three (2 %) cancer patients.

Withdrawal from Chronic Treatment

Approximately 50 % of cancer patients continued use of TTS fentanyl until death. Only 11 (7 %) withdrew from treatment because of inadequate pain control. While disease progression could not be documented in all cases, it probably contributed to intensified pain in this subset of patients. Adverse experiences accounted for the withdrawal of 13 (9 %) patients. Nausea and vomiting were cited as the reason for approximately half of these withdrawals. Multiple opioid-related side effects accounted for an additional three withdrawals during the first 7 weeks of therapy. None of these effects were considered serious. One additional patient withdrew because of bacterial sepsis and hypotension, and another had renal dysfunction and became comatose [11]; both were seriously ill from cancer at the time of study entry.

Adverse Experiences

TTS fentanyl was generally well-tolerated by the patients who used it chronically for cancer pain. Hypoventilation occurred in only three patients (2 %). The most frequently reported complaints were nausea (23 %) and vomiting (22 %). Other reactions reported for 10 % or more patients included constipation, dry mouth, somnolence, confusion, asthenia and sweating. In view of the advanced disease states and adjunctive treatments of these patients, the precise role of TTS fentanyl in causing these symptoms is uncertain.

Topical Effects

The topical effects observed during TTS fentanyl use have been minimal. Only 4 % of patients using TTS fentanyl have reported an application site reaction. There have been no complaints of sensitization. When skin sites were evaluated under double blind conditions in postoperative studies, the topical effects of TTS fentanyl could not be distinguished from those of transdermal placebos [Alza Corporation data].

Conclusion

The TTS fentanyl delivery profile can provide 72 h of pain control from a single dose, reduces the frequency of remedication, and promotes good compliance – all optimizing the opportunity to achieve good pain control. The simplicity of the TTS fentanyl regimen is a major advantage for both patients and caregivers.

References

1. v. Bormann B, Ratthey K, Schwetlick G, Schneider C, Muller H, Hempelmann G (1988) Transdermal fentanyl for postoperative pain control. Anasth Intensivther Notfallmed 23: 3–8
2. Caplan RA, Ready LB, Oden RV, Matsen III FA, Nessly ML, Olsson GL (1989) Transdermal fentanyl for postoperative pain management: a double-blind placebo study. JAMA 261 (7): 1036–1039
3. Coyle N, Adelhard J, Foley KM (1990) Characteristics of terminal illness in advanced cancer patients and other symptoms during the last four weeks of life. J Pain Symp Man (in press)
4. Duthie DJ, McLaren AD, Nimmo WS (1986) Pharmacokinetics of fentanyl during constant rate i.v. infusion for the relief of pain after surgery. Br J Anaesth 58: 950–956
5. Foley KM (1985) The treatment of cancer pain. New Engl J Med 313 (2): 85–95
6. Gourlay GK, Kowalski SR, Plummer JL, Cousins MJ, Armstrong PJ (1988) Fentanyl blood concentration-analgesic response relationship in the treatment of postoperative pain. Anesth Analg 67: 329–337
7. Holley FO, Steennis CV (1988) Postoperative analgesia with fentanyl: pharmacokinetics and pharmacodynamics of constant-rate i.v. and transdermal delivery. Br J Anaesth 60: 608–613
8. Larijani GE, Bell SD, Goldberg ME, Lessin JB (1988) Pharmacokinetics of fentanyl following transdermal application. Anesthesiology 69 (3A): A363
9. Latasch L, Luders S (1989) Transdermal fentanyl against postoperative pain. Acta Anaesthesiol Belg 40 (2): 113–119
10. McLeskey C, MacRae J (1990) Transdermal fentanyl for postoperative pain following lower abdominal surgery. Anesth Anal 70: S264
11. Miser AW, Narang PK, Dothage JA, Young RC, Sindelar W, Wiser JS (1989) Transdermal fentanyl for pain control in patients with cancer. Pain 37: 15–21
12. Nimmo WS, Todd JG (1985) Fentanyl by constant rate i.v. infusion for postoperative analgesia. Br J Anaesth 57: 250–254
13. Payne R, Moran K, Southam M (1990) The role of transdermal fentanyl in the management of cancer pain. In: Estafanous FG (ed) Opioids in Anesthesia. Butterworth-Heinemann Publishers, Chapter 21: 215–222
14. Plezia PM, Linford J, Kramer TH, Iacono RP, Hameroff SR (1988) Transdermally administered fentanyl for postoperative pain: a randomized, double-blind, placebo controlled trial. Anesthesiology 69 (3A): A364
15. Plezia PM, Kramer TH, Linford J, Hameroff SR (1989) Transdermal fentanyl: pharmacokinetics and preliminary clinical evaluation. Pharmacotherapy 9 (1): 2–9
16. Rowbotham DJ, Wyld R, Peacock JE, Duthie DJR, Nimmo WS (1989) Transdermal fentanyl for the relief of pain after upper abdominal surgery. Br J Anaesth 63: 56–59
17. Simmonds MA, Blain C, Richenbacher J, Southam MA, Hershey MS (1988) A new approach to the administration of opiates: TTS (fentanyl) in the management of pain in patients with cancer. J Pain Symptom Management 3 (3): S18
18. Varvel JR, Shafer SL, Hwang SS, Coen PA, Stanski DR (1989) Absorption characteristics of transdermally administered fentanyl. Anesthesiology 70: 928–934

Part IV. Postoperative Pain Management with TTS Fentanyl

Pharmacokinetics and Pharmacodynamics

G. K. Gourlay and L. E. Mather

Introduction

The theoretical background provided by L. E. Mather and G. K. Gourlay (this volume) indicated that the TTS fentanyl systems can provide a zero order input rate for at least 24 h that would mimic a constant rate intravenous infusion. In fact, the TTS fentanyl systems at a delivery rate of 100 μg/h have been shown to provide similar serum fentanyl concentrations at steady state to the intravenous infusion of fentanyl at an equivalent rate [6]. The currently available methods of treating postoperative pain have also been reviewed (Part 2). The continuous infusion of a number of opioids including morphine [18], pethidine [19] and fentanyl [14] has been shown to provide more reliable postoperative pain relief than that obtained from conventional intramuscular opioid regimens. However, there is at least a five-fold range of interpatient variability in the minimum effective blood opioid concentration (MEC) required to effectively control postoperative pain [2, 5, 8, 20]. Therefore, there are at least two possible approaches in the clinical implementation of zero order infusions to control postoperative pain. Firstly, the physician could use infusion rates which will provide steady-state blood opioid concentrations that are towards the higher end of the range of MECs, thereby providing acceptable pain relief to the majority of patients. The disadvantage of the approach is that the steady-state concentrations will still be inadequate for some patients while being excessive for a significant proportion of patients, probably causing unwanted and unpleasant side effects. The second approach is to attempt to individualize the infusion rate for each patient to maximize pain relief but minimize side effects.

We have conducted both open [9] and double blind (TTS fentanyl versus placebo) [10] evaluations of the TTS fentanyl system in the control of postoperative pain resulting from surgical procedures involving abdominal incisions. We elected to individualize the TTS fentanyl infusion rate by selecting the area of systems applied to each patient for two reasons: (a) we believed this to be the most desirable approach, and (b) concurrent studies [6, 11, 17, 21] intended to use a constant TTS fentanyl infusion rate, invariably, 100 μg/h. This chapter reviews the pharmacokinetics and pharmacodynamic effects from both the open und double blind studies of TTS fentanyl in the treatment of postoperative pain.

Study Design

Patients

Patients were aged between 18 and 70 years and were scheduled to have surgery involving an abdominal incision. Patients with significantly impaired hepatic or renal function, a chronic respiratory illness, documented hypersensitivity to opioids or a history of drug abuse were excluded from the study. Thirteen patients were included in an open study examining pharmacokinetics and pharmacodynamics of the TTS fentanyl systems while forty patients were entered into the double blind comparison of pain relief and side effects of TTS fentanyl ($n = 20$) and placebo ($n = 20$) systems.

Psychometric Tests Prior to Surgery

Prior to surgery, each patient completed the following psychometric tests which were required to calculate the area of TTS fentanyl to be applied to individual patients (see below "Calculation of the Dose Rate ..."):

1. The *Illness Behaviour Questionnaire,* which scores seven traits useful in the examination of the impact of the surgical event on the patient [15]
2. The *Beck Depression Inventory,* a self-rating scale of depression [3]
3. The *Eysenck Personality Questionnaire,* which examines extroversion/introversion, neuroticism and social conformity (i.e., the tendency for the patient to answer questions to please the investigator rather than truthfully) [7]

Anesthetic Technique

Patients were premedicated with oral diazepam and anesthesia was induced with thiopentone. Muscle relaxation for endotracheal intubation was facilitated with suxamethonium. Anesthesia was maintained with nitrous oxide/oxygen, pancuronium, and enflurane if required. Patients who had TTS fentanyl systems in situ had intraoperative intravenous fentanyl (2 μg/kg) administered while those patients who had placebo systems in situ received pethidine (1 mg/kg) instead of the fentanyl. This was achieved using precoded syringes, thereby preserving the double blind nature of the study design. The intraoperative administration of pethidine (25 mg intravenous increments) was allowed only if the anesthetist judged that the patient required additional opioid analgesia rather than increasing the depth of anesthesia with enflurane.

Calculation of the Dose Rate (Area) of TTS Fentanyl To Be Applied to Each Patient

We elected to individualize the dose rate for each patient in an attempt to provide optimal postoperative pain relief. A previous study [8] had investigated the blood concentration-analgesic response relationship of fentanyl incorporated in a patient-controlled analgesia (PCA) infusion device. The patients underwent similar surgical procedures to those of patients participating in TTS fentanyl studies. Multiple linear regression analysis with either mean hourly fentanyl demand rate or MEC for fentanyl as the independent variable and a range of anthropometric measurements and the results of the preoperative psychometric tests (see above, "Psychometric Tests Prior to Surgery") as dependent variables resulted in the following equation:

$$\text{dose rate} = 71 - 5 \cdot \text{IBQ1} + 9 \cdot \text{IBQ2} - 15 \cdot \text{SEX}$$

where dose rate is the hourly fentanyl input rate (μg/h), IBQ1 and IBQ2 are the first (general hypochondriasis) and second (disease conviction) factors of the Illness Behaviour Questionnaire respectively, and SEX represents 1 for males and 2 for females. The nominal dose rate applied was adjusted to the available dose rates, either 25, 50, 75, 100 or 125 μg/h (i.e., 10, 20, 30, 40, or 50 cm^2 respectively). The most commonly used dose rates were 50 or 75 μg/h. Inspection of the above equation revealed that females required an approximately 25% lower fentanyl dose rate which was most likely due to a subtle pharmacokinetic difference between the sexes [8]. This equation was used preoperatively using the patient's scores on IBQ1 and IBQ2 to calculate the dose rate.

Period of Application of the TTS Fentanyl Systems

The required area of TTS fentanyl (or placebo) systems was applied to a nonhairy area of the upper anterior chest wall of each patient following induction of anesthesia and within 10 min of the intraoperative intravenous opioid (i.e., either fentanyl (active) or pethidine (placebo)) loading dose. At the time that these studies were designed, we were unaware of the prolonged period before effective fentanyl concentrations would be achieved from the TTS fentanyl systems (see below). Each system remained in situ for exactly 24 h; it was then removed and an equivalent area applied to an identical site on the contralateral side and left in situ for a further 24 h after which time it was removed. There were no alterations to the area of TTS systems applied for day 1 and day 2 in the double blind study. However, in the open study, three patients required reductions in the area applied due to respiratory depression (assessed by respiratory rate) while one patient required an increase in area applied due to inadequate pain relief.

Supplementary Pain Relief and Antiemetic Therapy

Throughout the 48 h period following TTS system application, additional analgesic medication was available on patient request by the administration of intravenous bolus doses of pethidine (25–50 mg), depending on the clinical assessment of the patient (by one of our research nurses), provided that the unstimulated respiratory rate was greater than 10 breaths/min and there were no signs of significant CNS depression. Metoclopramide (10 mg intravenously) was administered as required for the symptomatic relief of nausea and vomiting.

Clinical Monitoring of Patients

The patients in this study were under continuous observation by the research nursing staff from Flinders Medical Centre's pain management unit for the first 48 h postoperatively. Blood pressure, pulse, and respiratory rate were measured hourly for the duration of the study. In addition, visual analogue pain scores (VAPS) and sedation rating scores (SRS) were obtained hourly except between 2400 and 0600, when they were obtained hourly only if the patient was awake. The SRS was a categorical scale of 1–5 where 1 represents awake, 2 drowsy, 3 dozing, 4 sleeping, and 5 awake only when roused.

Blood Sampling and Analysis of Blood Fentanyl Concentrations

Blood samples were collected frequently during the first hour following the intravenous fentanyl dose and thereafter at hourly intervals for 48 h. The concentration of fentanyl in the blood samples was quantitated by gas-liquid chromatography with nitrogen-phosphorus detection [12]. The standard curve was linear, passed through the origin and had a lower limit of detection of 0.1 ng/ml.

Pharmacokinetic Analysis

Inspection of the various blood fentanyl concentration time curves indicated that there was a delay time, which varied between patients, before clinically significant blood fentanyl concentrations were achieved. We have previously documented that the mean MEC for fentanyl was 0.63 ng/ml in a group of patients undergoing surgical procedures involving abdominal incisions. Therefore, we have arbitrarily defined the *delay time* as the length of time between TTS fentanyl application and the earlier of two consecutive blood fentanyl concentrations exceeding 0.63 ng/ml [9]. Similarly, following system removal, there was a delay before the blood fentanyl concentration fell significantly. We have termed this the *decay time,* and we defined it as the time between removal and the moment when the blood fentanyl concentration falls below 0.63 ng/ml.

Pharmacokinetic Aspects

The anthropometric data, types of operation, intravenous opioid doses, dose rates applied, and delay and decay times are given in Table 1 for patients entered into the open study of efficacy. Patients with a similar age and weight range and type of surgical procedure were entered in the double blind study.

The blood fentanyl concentration-time profiles from patients having low (patient 13), intermediate (patient 1) and high (patient 3) 36–48 h blood fentanyl concentrations (i.e., "steady state" concentrations) are shown in Fig. 1. The fentanyl dose rates were 75 μg/h for patients 1 and 3 and 50 μg/h for patient 13. Similar profiles were obtained from patients with TTS fentanyl systems applied in the double blind study. The data in Fig. 1 clearly show three phases: 1. a delay time, 2. an apparent steady state in the last 12 h period of each 24 h dosing interval, and 3. a decay time after removal of the TTS fentanyl systems.

The Delay Time

Figure 1 clearly shows that there is a delay from the time of TTS fentanyl system application to the attainment of effective blood fentanyl concentrations. The delay time is difficult to define in individual patients without actually measuring blood fentanyl concentrations. We arbitrarily defined the delay time, taking the critical blood fentanyl concentration as 0.6 ng/ml, which was the mean MEC for fentanyl in a PCA study (MEC range was 0.2–1.2 ng/ml) using a similar range of surgical procedures in a similar patient group to that used for this study [8]. Under these circumstances, the delay time ranged from 1.2 h to 31.3 h, with a mean value of 12.7 h (Table 1) and was noted to be quite variable between patients. Using the same methodology, the mean (± SD) delay time was 16.7 ± 10.0 h in the double blind study (Table 2). The mean delay time was 10.1 ± 5.7 and 18.9 ± 10.9 for the most frequently used dose rates of 75 μg/h and 50 μg/ respectively. At least two other studies [16, 21] have reported similar results. Varvel et al. [21] have performed studies where serum fentanyl concentrations were quantitated following both intravenous and transdermal doses in the same patient, allowing a definitive calculation of absorption rate into the systemic circulation (using the Loo-Riegelman method). The area of TTS fentanyl system applied was 40 cm^2, providing a nominal input rate of 100 μg/h. The results indicated that the systemic absorption rate was very low in the 0–4 h period, increased during the 4–8 h period, and remained relatively constant, with a mean value of 92 μg/h (coefficient of variation = 28%) from 8 to 24 h. There is agreement between various reports [6, 9–11, 16, 17, 21] concerning the probable reason for the delay time which results from the time taken to establish a reservoir of fentanyl in the stratum corneum. Therefore, these data indicated that, while there is a definite delay time, its actual magnitude

Table 1. Patient characteristics, operations performed, delay time, decay time and transdermal- and bolus fentanyl doses used

Patient	Sex	Age (years)	Weight (kg)	Operation	Fentanyl bolus (µg)	Transdermal fentanyl dose (µg/hd)		Delay time* (h)	Decay time** (h)
						Day 1	Day 2		
1	F	33	84.5	Partial hepatectomy	200	75	75	8.0	21.5
2	F	24	63.0	Cholecystectomy	150	100	125	4.0	> 21.2[a]
3	F	30	59.4	Cholecystectomy	150	75	50	1.2	> 22.5[a]
4	M	30	74.0	Highly selective vagotomy	100	75	75	8.0	11.75
5	F	20	82.2	Cholecystectomy	200	75	50	40	24.9
6	F	51	76.0	Cholecystectomy	200	50	50	31.25	2.25
7	M	58	88.8	Colostomy takedown	100	75	75	9.2	8.1
8	F	57	78.9	Excision of bowel tumor	200	75	75	18.0	15.5
9	M	65	78.0	Pseudomyxoma drain	200	75	75	15.3	21.4
10	M	68	86.5	Cholecystectomy	200	75	75	18.2	> 14.4[a]
11	M	33	57.0	Laparotomy	200	75	50	9.0	16.5
12	F	29	53.0	Cholecystectomy	200	75	75	8.0	22.75
13	F	68	51.5	Right hemicolectomy	100	50	50	30.5	6.75
Mean	8F/5M	44	71		170			12.7	16.1
SD		18	12.4		43			9.6	7.1
Median						75	75		

* The latency between patch application and the time taken to reach a blood fentanyl concentration of 0.63 ng/ml which was the mean fentanyl MEC for a similar range of operations to that studied in this communication.

** The latency from 48 h (when TTS Fentanyl systems were removed) until the blood fentanyl concentration falls below 0.63 ng/ml.

a Blood fentanyl concentration had not fallen below 0.63 ng/ml at time of last sample.

Table 2. Delay times, mean blood fentanyl concentrations for the 12–24 and 36–48 h time periods and nominal hourly dose rates in the patients treated with TTS Fentanyl in the double blind study

Patient No.	Delay time** (h)	Mean fentanyl concentrations (ng/ml) 12–24 h			36–48 h			Nominal dose rate (μg/h)
		Mean	SD	*n**	Mean	SD	*n**	
2	29.8	0.40	0.10	12	0.95	0.10	11	50
4	9.0	1.00	0.20	12	1.25	0.10	12	50
5	10.0	1.05	0.20	11	0.90	0.15	11	50
6	26.1	0.40	0.15	10	0.75	0.15	12	25
9	7.2	1.10	0.10	9	1.90	0.15	12	75
12	27.0	0.45	0.15	12	0.90	0.05	10	25
14	28.4	0.55	0.10	12	1.30	0.25	12	50
15	10.8	1.10	0.20	12	1.80	0.20	11	50
16	4.9	1.30	0.15	11	2.05	0.15	12	50
17	17.1	0.70	0.35	12	0.70	0.15	13	50
22	18.0	0.70	0.50	10	1.10	0.25	12	75
25	8.5	1.05	0.35	12	2.10	0.70	11	50
27[a]	—	—	—	—	—	—	—	75
28	8.0	0.95	0.10	12	1.30	0.15	12	50
29	3.0	1.95	0.20	12	2.40	0.30	11	75
31	27.9	0.45	0.10	12	0.85	0.10	12	50
34	14.3	1.05	0.20	11	1.90	0.15	13	75
35	20.5	0.65	0.25	12	1.45	0.25	12	50
38	37.3	0.35	0.10	12	0.55	0.15	12	50
39	10.2	1.00	0.15	13	1.65	0.25	12	50
Mean	16.7	0.85			1.36			
SD	10.0	0.40			0.55			

* n = number of blood fentanyl concentrations in each 12 h period.
** Defined in Table 1.
a Patient No. 27 had an interfering peak such that blood fentanyl concentrations could not reliably be determined. Therefore, delay time and mean fentanyl concentrations are not shown.

depends on the criteria used in its definition. In contrast to the wide variability in the pharmacokinetic parameters describing fentanyl disposition (see Mather and Gourlay, this volume) there is excellent reproducibility in the actual blood (serum) fentanyl concentration time curves between the various studies concerning transdermal fentanyl. Thus, if effective fentanyl blood concentrations are required in the immediate postoperative period, the TTS fentanyl systems should be applied 12–18 h prior to surgery. Further, the systems could be expected to provide acceptable "premedication" conditions as the fentanyl blood concentration would slowly rise over this period to sedate and relax the patient prior to surgery.

Pseudo Steady State

Figure 1 shows that there was a pseudo steady state after approximately 12 h from TTS fentanyl system application. The data in Table 2 from the double blind study provide representative information from our patients which is consistent with other published reports where TTS fentanyl systems were left in situ for 24 h. However, while most studies terminated the study at 24 h, we changed the TTS systems at this point and studied the patients for a further 24 h [9, 10]. It is apparent (Fig. 1 and Table 2) that the blood fentanyl concentrations continued to increase after 24 h such that the mean 36–48 h blood fentanyl concentrations were significantly greater than the 12–24 h values (paired Student's *t* test). Figure 2 shows the mean 36–48 h fentanyl concentration (for all patients) as a function of the TTS fentanyl dose rate and

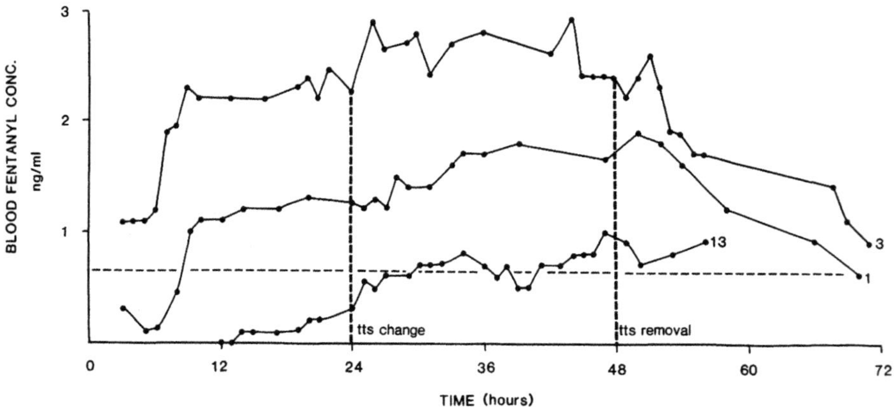

Fig. 1. Blood fentanyl concentration (ng/ml) as a function of time (h), following the application of TTS Fentanyl systems intraoperatively. Patients 3, 13 and 1 had the highest, lowest and an intermediate mean 36–48 h blood fentanyl concentration respectively. TTS change represents the time at which the systems were changed (i.e., 24 h) while TTS removal represents the time when the second lot of systems were removed. The line parallel to the x-axis represents the mean minimum effective concentration for fentanyl (0.63 ng/ml) to control postoperative pain [8]

indicates there is a significant ($P < 0.05$) linear relationship between steady state fentanyl concentration and dose (i.e., infusion rate). This relationship also helps to explain why the delay time to reach effective blood fentanyl concentrations is shorter as the dose rate increases (see above). The mean 12–24 h blood fentanyl concentrations normalized for an input rate of 25 μg/h (i.e., 0.31 ng/ml) obtained in our studies were lower than the dose-normalized values found at 24 h (i.e., 0.5–0.6 ng/ml) following a constant rate intravenous infusion varying from 25–100 μg/h [14], probably as a consequence of true steady state blood concentrations not being achieved within the 12–24 h period. However, the mean 36–48 h blood fentanyl concentrations normalized per 25 μg/h dose rate (0.5 ng/ml) were consistent with those from the equivalent intravenous rate, indicating steady state conditions.

More recent studies where the same TTS fentanyl systems (75 μg/h) were left in situ for 72 h have revealed a slightly different profile (data on file, ALZA Corporation). In this situation, the pseudo steady state was maintained for at least 60 h and the mean 36–48 h fentanyl concentrations

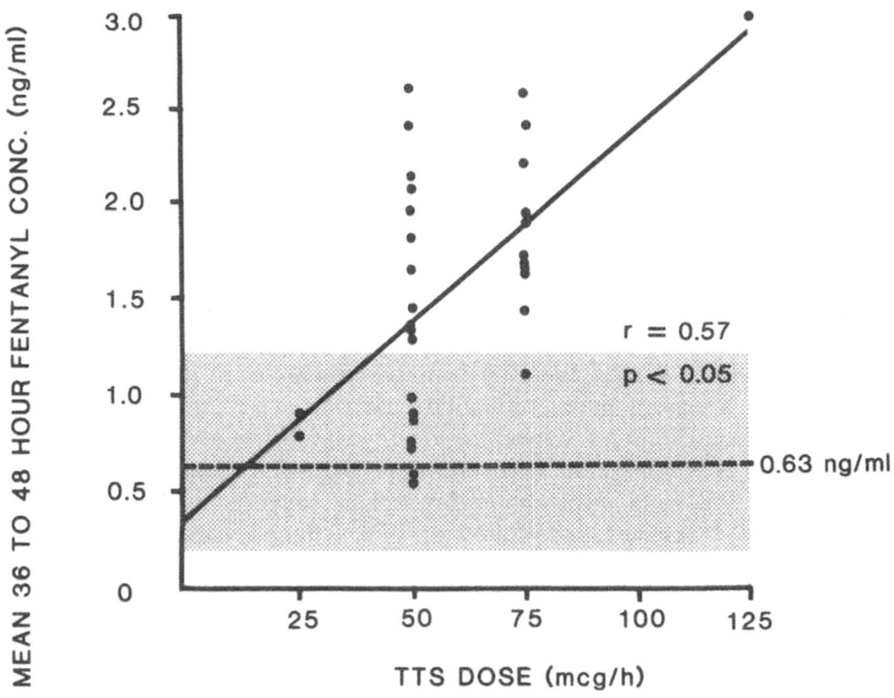

Fig. 2. Mean 36–48 h blood fentanyl concentration (ng/ml) as a function of TTS Fentanyl dose /μg/h). Each point in the graph represents an individual patient. The dashed line at 0.63 ng/ml represents the mean MEC for fentanyl to control postoperative pain obtained in a similar group of patients [8] in whom fentanyl was administered in a PCA infusion pump. The shaded area around this dashed line represents the extremes in MEC values for fentanyl obtained in the PCA study

were similar to the 12–24 h concentrations. The reason for the discrepancy between the two studies is not immediately clear, but a possible explanation may relate to differences in the delay and decay times (see below) where the latter is probably longer than the former.

In all but two patients, the blood fentanyl concentrations exceeded the critical value of 0.63 ng/ml, and those two patients were very close to this arbitrary level (Fig. 2). However, the shaded adrea represents the extremes of the MEC for fentanyl obtained from the PCA study [8]. Clearly, dose rates of at least 75 μg/h would be required to provide acceptable analgesia in the majority of patients. The mean (± SD) 36–48 h blood fentanyl concentrations were 1.85 (± 0.72) ng/ml and 1.36 (± 0.55) ng/ml in the open- and double blind studies respectively. The lower level in the double blind study occurred because of the greater proportion of patients with an input rate of 50 μg/h. Collectively, these data suggest that the TTS fentanyl systems have the potential to provide significant postoperative analgesia in the majority of patients, but it may take longer than 24 h to achieve satisfactory analgesia if they are applied at the time of surgery. Alternative pain-relieving procedures will inevitably be required under these conditions. Further, physicians should be aware of this delay if they decide to increase the TTS fentanyl dose because of inadequate analgesia.

Decay Time

Figure 1 also shows that the blood fentanyl concentrations decrease very slowly once the TTS fentanyl systems have been removed. We defined the decay time in an analogous manner to the initial delay time, i.e., as the time between removal of the TTS fentanyl system and the time for the blood fentanyl concentration to fall below 0.63 ng/ml. The mean (± SD) decay time was 16.1 (± 7.1) h with a range of 2.3 to > 22.2 h. Holley and van Steennis [11] and Duthie et al. [6] calculated a terminal half-life for fentanyl of approximately 16 h after the TTS fentanyl systems were removed. In our studies, the apparent mean total body clearance (i.e., theoretical input rate/mean blood fentanyl concentration for the 36–48 h period) was 721 ml/min, which is consistent with literature reports for fentanyl clearance determined following intravenous doses. This suggests that the elevated blood fentanyl concentrations following TTS fentanyl system removal were not a consequence of low fentanyl clearance. Rather, it suggests that the previously proposed reservoir of fentanyl in the skin slowly washes out, thereby maintaining the blood fentanyl concentrations. Further and more precise evidence to support this concept has been provided by a study in which fentanyl pharmacokinetics were estimated following both intravenous and transdermal doses in the same surgical patients [21]. The mean terminal half-life following TTS fentanyl system removal was estimated to be 17 h, while that following intravenous fentanyl averaged 6.1 h.

The clinical significance of this prolonged decay phase are two-fold. Firstly, the beneficial effect of effective pain control could continue for 12–24 h after the TTS fentanyl systems have been removed. This needs to be interpreted in the knowledge of a reducing postoperative stimulus during this time, particularly if the systems are removed 48 h postoperatively. Secondly, adverse effects could also continue for a longer than expected time based on normal fentanyl pharmacokinetics. Hence, removing the TTS fentanyl systems will not immediately result in the elimination of adverse effects and more than a single naloxone dose could possibly be required in some cases.

Pharmacodynamic Effects

Figures 3, 4 show sedation scores, respiratory rate, pain intensity scores, and blood fentanyl concentrations as a function of time for two patients who represent different pharmacodynamic aspects of the TTS fentanyl systems. The lower panels (Figs. 3 and 4) showing the blood fentanyl concentrations are displayed using the more traditional logarithimic Y axis (unlike Fig. 1 where a linear axis is used) and this representation emphasizes the pseudo steady state aspect of TTS fentanyl pharmacokinetics, particularly for patient 5 (Fig. 3). The mean 36–48 h steady state concentration for patients 5 and 10 (from the open study) were 2.4 and 1.4 ng/ml respectively.

Pain Intensity Scores

The pain scores for both patients showed wide fluctuations throughout the study period although the fluctuations were more frequent for patient 5. This patient had periods of adequate pain control (low pain scores) usually during the night and periods of less adequate pain control (usually during the day) although the mean pseudo steady state blood fentanyl concentration was among the highest recorded (2.4 ng/ml) and was not different between the periods of adequate and inadequate pain control. These higher pain scores were associated with specific incidents (such as mobilization, chest physiotherapy, etc.) which would be expected to be more painful. Additional intravenous analgesia was requested but refused because of the low respiratory rate. Patient 10 showed much less fluctuation in pain scores and required overall less pethidine supplementation despite having a much lower steady-state blood fentanyl concentration (1.4 ng/ml).

However, Table 3 shows the mean pain intensity scores for the TTS fentanyl and TTS placebo groups subdivided into 12 h time intervals. There was no significant difference (analysis of variance) between the TTS fentanyl and TTS placebo groups, nor was there a significant treatment by time interaction, indicating that the scores followed the same trend in both groups. It should be noted that all patients required at least one dose of supplementary intravenous pethidine (see below). Therefore, we concluded that the quality of pain relief was similar between the fentanyl and placebo groups

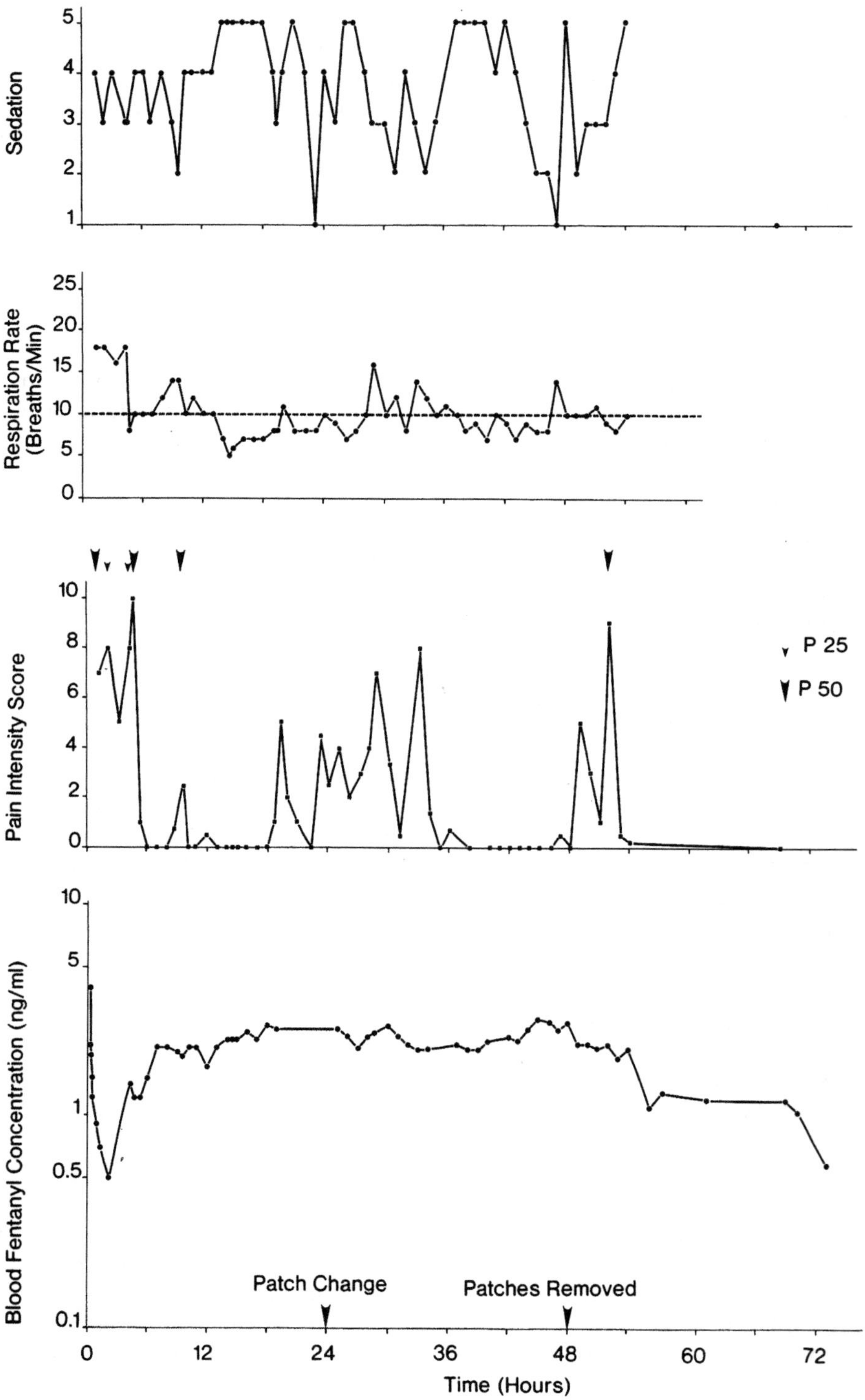

Sedation
5
4
3
2
1
Respiration Rate (Breaths/Min)
25
20
15
10
5
0
Pain Intensity Score
10
8
6
4
2
0
P 25
P 50
Blood Fentanyl Concentration (ng/ml)
10
5
1
0.5
0.1
Patch Change
Patches Removed
0
12
24
36
48
60
72
Time (Hours)

Table 3. Mean pain intensity scores for the TTS-Fentanyl- and TTS-placebo-treated patients throughout the 48 h study period

Time (h)	TTS Fentanyl patients*		TTS placebo patients*	
	Mean	SD	Mean	SD
0–12	3.84	2.13	4.06	2.41
12–24	2.46	1.24	2.98	1.93
24–36	2.28	1.43	3.00	2.07
36–48	1.83	1.69	2.26	1.57

* There was no significant difference between pain scores in the two groups, as assessed by an analysis of variance

where additional intravenous analgesia was available "on demand" via our research nurses.

Supplementary or Additional Analgesia

Figs. 3 and 4 show that these two patients, like all patients in both the open and double blind studies, required additional intravenous pethidine which was greatest in the 0–12 h period. We have grouped the pethidine supplementation into 12 h time periods (e.g., 0–12, 12–24, etc.) for statistical analysis. In the open study there was a significantly greater ($P < 0.001$, Friedman's test) requirement for pethidine supplementation in the 0–12 h time (129 ± 79 mg) period than in the 12–24 h (39 ± 74 mg), 24–36 h (39 ± 35 mg) and 36–48 h (27 ± 44 mg pethidine) time periods. In the double blind study, there was no significant difference between the fentanyl and placebo groups in the 0–12 h time period, but significantly less ($P < 0.05$) pethidine was required by patients in the TTS fentanyl group than by those in the TTS placebo group in the 12–24, 24–36 and 36–48 h periods (Table 4).

The extent of pethidine supplementation in the TTS fentanyl group was approximately half that of the placebo group when there was a significant difference between the two groups. The high level of pethidine supplementation in the TTS fentanyl group in the 0–12 h time period is consistent with the pharmacokinetic finding (Fig. 1, Tables 1 and 2) of a long delay time of approximately 12 h before clinically significant blood fentanyl concentrations are achieved from the TTS fentanyl systems. There was no correlation (Spearman's rank correlation) between supplementary pethidine requirements and mean 36–48 h blood fentanyl concentration. The level of pethidine

◀ **Fig. 3.** Blood fentanyl concentration, visual analogue pain scores, respiratory rates, and sedation rating scores in patient 5, in whom there was significant bradypnea during the postoperative period. The large and small arrows beside P50 and P25 represent the times when supplementary pethidine, 50 mg and 25 mg respectively, were administered. The categorical scale for the sedation rating score is given in the study design section

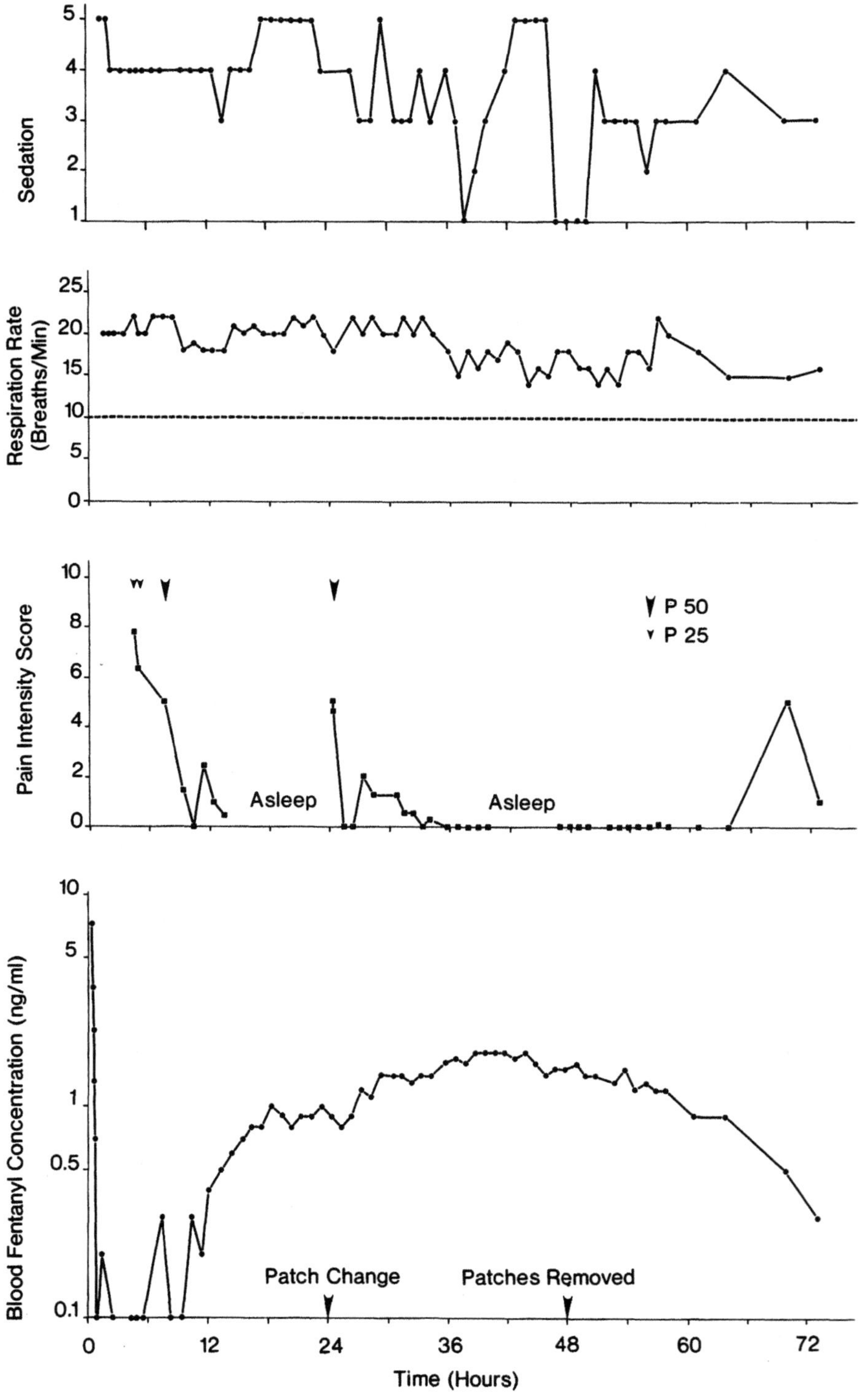
Sedation
Respiration Rate (Breaths/Min)
Pain Intensity Score
P 50
P 25
Asleep
Asleep
Blood Fentanyl Concentration (ng/ml)
Patch Change
Patches Removed
Time (Hours)

Table 4. Supplementary pethidine requirements for patients in the TTS Fentanyl and TTS placebo groups

Time period	Supplementary pethidine requirements (mg) (mean ± SD) TTS Fentanyl group	Placebo group*	Significance**
0–12	216 ± 85	183 ± 84	*NS*
12–24	98 ± 77	162 ± 84	$P < 0.05$
24–36	82 ± 77	162 ± 93	$P < 0.05$
36–48	66 ± 74	125 ± 91	$P < 0.05$
Total	461 ± 274	617 ± 289	*NS*

* Excludes the intraoperative pethidine dose in patients in the TTS placebo group.
** Indicates whether a difference in pethidine requirements could be detected between patients in the TTS Fentanyl and TTS placebo groups in each 12 h time period – Student's *t* test for unpaired observations.

supplementation in the placebo group was similar for the four time periods (Table 4). There was no significant difference between the TTS fentanyl and placebo groups in the total amount of pethidine supplementation because of the pronounced influence of the level of supplementation from the 0–12 h period to the total amount. In fact, proportionally more of the total pethidine supplementation was administered to the TTS fentanyl group than the placebo group (47% compared to 30%) during the 0–12 h time period. While this may reflect the longer duration of pain relief associated with intraoperative pethidine compared to fentanyl, it is also consistent with the attainment of clinically effective blood fentanyl concentrations after the initial delay. Therefore, the interpretation of the pain scores and pethidine supplementation data together indicates that the TTS fentanyl systems are efficacious in the control of postoperative pain following abdominal surgical procedures.

Sedation

Figures 3 and 4 show the sedation rating scores (upper panel) as a function of time, where 1 represents awake and 5 represents awake only when roused. It is apparent that the sedation scores varied between these two extremes with a predominance of scores between 3 (dozing) and 4 (mostly sleeping). Table 5

◀ **Fig. 4.** Blood fentanyl concentration, visual analogue pain scores, respiratory rates, and sedation rating scores in patient 10, who represents the usual respiratory pattern in the postoperative period with the TTS Fentanyl systems. The large and small *arrows* beside P50 and P25 represent the times when supplementary pethidine, 50 mg and 25 mg respectively, were administered

Table 5. Mean sedation scores for the TTS Fentanyl and TTS placebo treated patients throughout the 48 h study period

Time (h)	TTS Fentanyl patients*		TTS placebo patients*	
	Mean	SD	Mean	SD
0–12*	3.67	0.55	4.05	0.51
12–24	3.19	0.79	3.36	0.70
24–36*	2.40	0.73	2.20	0.56
36–48	3.17	0.70	3.02	0.53

There was no significant difference between sedation scores in the two groups as assessed by analysis of variance.
* These time periods generally correspond to daylight hours.

gives the mean sedation scores for the TTS fentanyl and placebo groups in the double blind study. There was no significant difference between the two groups as assessed by analysis of variance, nor was there a significant treatment by time interaction indicating that the scores followed similar trends in both groups. This finding is not unexpected as it must be interpreted in the light of the fact that all patients received additional intravenous pethidine which was available essentially on demand to optimize pain relief. In the double blind study, patients in the TTS fentanyl group required significantly less pethidine because of the contribution of fentanyl. Nevertheless, both fentanyl and pethidine would contribute to sedation scores as well as the other subjective side effects.

Respiratory Depression

The respiratory rate (breaths/min) measured every hour as a function of time are shown for two patients with TTS fentanyl systems in situ. One patient (Fig. 4) had an adequate respiratory pattern throughout the 72 h of the study while the other patient (Fig. 3) had respiratory rates which gave cause for concern. We chose a level of concern to be that of two consecutive respiratory rate measurements of less than 10 breaths/min. We elected to use the regular assessment of respiratory rate as the index of potential respiratory depression because this measurement is almost universally undertaken in the postoperative period. The low respiratory rates for the patient shown in Fig. 3 (in the open study) were associated with high mean pseudo steady state blood fentanyl concentrations (2.4 ng/ml) and with no pethidine supplementation after 10 h while the TTS fentanyl systems were in situ. It is apparent that the pain intensity scores were periodically high throughout this period and the patient made frequent requests for additional analgesia which were refused because of our concern regarding her respiratory status. The TTS fentanyl dose was reduced from 75 to 50 μg/h at 14.5 h and supplemental oxygen was administered for 15 h. The patient recovered without ill effect. The common features to all three patients with low respiratory rates were

a) mean pseudo steady state blood fentanyl concentration of greater than 2 ng/ml, a level which has been demonstrated to result in respiratory depression as shown by a shift to the right in the carbon dioxide response curves [1, 4], and
b) minimal total pethidine supplementation (between 100 and 250 mg which was administered in the 0–12 h time period).

The respiratory depression usually occurred in the 12–24 and 24–36 h time periods. These findings implicate the fentanyl from the TTS fentanyl systems as the major cause of this side effect. However, all three patients recovered uneventfully and no patient in the double blind study was classified (by our definition) as having respiratory depression, although three patients had isolated readings below 10 breaths/min. Therefore, the overall incidence of respiratory depression was 3 out of 33 (13 in open study and 20 in double blind study) or 9% of patients. However, it should be noted that respiratory depression is a potential consequence of any opioid analgesic technique and was noted in one-third of patients having a postoperative continuous infusion of fentanyl at a rate of 125 µ/h [11]. These authors also noted that ventilatory rates were unhelpful in detecting hypercapnia.

Incidence of Nausea

In the double blind study, 18 patients in the TTS fentanyl group and 15 patients in the TTS placebo group required metoclopramide for nausea (Table 6). The mean (± SD) metoclopramide doses over 48 h for patients in the TTS fentanyl and TTS placebo groups were 40 (± 25) mg and 27 (± 26) mg respectively. These differences were not significantly different.

Other Side Effects

There was a similar profile of side effects in patients receiving TTS fentanyl and TTS placebo systems (Table 6). One important consideration unique to the TTS systems rather than the opioid contained within the systems would be the incidence and severity of topical reactions as a consequence of the adhesive used to hold the systems tightly to the skin. Five patients in the TTS fentanyl and three patients in the TTS placebo group had an erythematous reaction in the area of skin occluded by the systems when assessed 1 h after the systems were removed. However, the majority of the erythema had disappeared when the area was reassessed at 6 h and the severity was considered only mild. Two patients had pruritis in the area occluded by TTS fentanyl systems. The dermatological side effects of the TTS fentanyl systems were considered very minor in those patients who experienced them. Other side effects reported by both groups of patients included headache, sedation and urinary retention and these effects could have been cause by either fentanyl or pethidine or a combination of both.

Table 6. Incidence of adverse effects in patients treated with TTS Fentanyl and TTS placebo systems

Side effect	No. of patients with adverse effects	
	TTS Fentanyl*	TTS placebo*
Nausea	18	15
Erythema	5	3
Urinary retention	3	3
Headache	2	1
Sedation	2	1
Dizziness	2	—
Pruritis	2	—
Pulmonary edema	1	—
Jerking hand and foot movements	1	—

* Twenty patients were randomly assigned to each group

Summary

Two questions must be considered when assessing the potential application of any new drug or technique:
a) is it efficacious?
b) are the incidence and severity of side effects acceptable?

Our studies described in this chapter attempted to address both questions using a study design that satisfied the requirements of scientific enquiry as well as those of optimal patient management.

The rationale underlying the use of TTS fentanyl systems is that relatively constant blood fentanyl concentrations will be produced which exceed the MEC and lead to relatively constant pain relief. This rationale has been verified in the treatment of postoperative pain where the efficacy of continuous infusions of fentanyl [11, 14] and other opioids such as morphine [5] and pethidine [2, 20] has already been established, as has that of fentanyl administered by PCA devices [8, 13]. For each of these opioids, a relationship between blood (plasma) opioid concentration and postoperative pain relief has been established. Therefore, there is considerable experimental evidence to support the rationale of the TTS fentanyl systems.

There is good agreement between the studies conducted in various centers throughout the world which examined the pharmacokinetic characteristics of the TTS fentanyl systems. The majority of these studies have identified the same three main characteristics, namely
a) a delay time before effective blood fentanyl concentrations are obtained,
b) pseudo steady state levels which are linearly related to the dose rate, and

c) a greater than expected time for the blood fentanyl concentration to fall substantially following TTS fentanyl system removal, which we have termed the decay time.

While all studies have identified the delay time, there is some debate as to the appropriate extent or duration of the delay time. The delay time of between 9–12 h reported in our studies for the more common dose rates of 50 or 75 μg/h are in agreement with the studies of Holley and van Steennis [11] and Varvel et al. [21] employing a dose rate of 100 μg/h although it should be noted that some patients had much longer delay times. In our studies, there appeared to be an inverse relationship between dose rate (25–100 μ/h) and delay time. The delay time need not be considered a disadvantage as it can be overcome by applying the systems prior to surgery; we would recommend at least 12 h before the expected induction of anesthesia. In fact, it is possible that the systems could provide acceptable premedication conditions as the slowly increasing blood fentanyl concentrations should provide a calm patient without the requirement for injected opioid or anxiolytic premedication. While the levels of blood fentanyl concentrations would be insufficient to provide ideal anesthesic conditions for surgery, they would provide acceptable baseline levels which could be easily supplemented intraoperatively. On emergence from anesthesia, the patient should have blood fentanyl concentrations to provide acceptable postoperative analgesia. There is uniform agreement between the different studies that the TTS fentanyl systems provide steady-state blood fentanyl concentrations after approximately 12–15 h which are in the previously documented [11, 13, 14] analgesic range for fentanyl (1–2 ng/ml at 24 h for an intravenous infusion of 100 μg/h).

The only study designed to allow a calculation of absorption rate and transdermal bioavailability has been undertaken by Varvel et al. [21]. These authors showed

a) that absorption rate was less than half the nominal rate (100 μg/h) up to 4 h
b) that the absorption rate increased during the period from 4–8 h, and
c) that after 8 h there was a relatively constant mean (± SD) absorption rate of 92 (± 26) μg/h.

However, the authors noted a large interpatient variability in absorption rate at steady state, within the range 80–115 μ/h. The transdermal bioavailability assessed by both model independent and model dependent (3 compartment Loo-Riegelman) methods was 92% ± 35%.

The following hypothesis is consistent with all these experimental findings. It is probable that a depot of fentanyl forms in the skin under the TTS fentanyl system. It takes some time for this depot to contain sufficient fentanyl to release to the systemic circulation and provide significant fentanyl concentrations because of the combined effects of the rate control membrane in the TTS system and the relatively impermeable barrier of the stratum corneum. This represents the delay time. An equilibrium is established where the release of fentanyl from the TTS system maintains a pseudo steady state. The rate of fentanyl absorption becomes zero order after 8 h but pseudo steady state is not reached until some time later, in accordance with general pharmacokinetic principles. True steady state is not achieved until 24–36 h. The depot continues to release fentanyl to the systemic circulation after the TTS system has been removed, thereby explaining the difference in fentanyl half-life between transdermal and intravenous administration in the same patients. In fact, Plezia et al. [16] have shown that up to 30% of the total dose absorbed remains contained within the skin reservoir at the time when the TTS fentanyl systems are removed.

The double blind study demonstrated the clinical efficacy of the TTS fentanyl systems where the patients in the group having TTS fentanyl systems in situ required approximately half the level of pethidine supplementation as the placebo group. There was no significant difference in pain intensity scores or sedation scores between the two groups. These results verify the findings of Rowbotham et al. [17], where the TTS fentanyl group required two-thirds the amount of morphine supplementation as the placebo group.

There was no significant difference between the TTS fentanyl and placebo groups with respect to side effects; these included nausea, sedation, headache and urinary retention. The dermatological effects of the TTS systems are minor. Our studies indicate that physicians could expect up to 9% of patients treated with TTS fentanyl to undergo a reduction of respiratory rate to a level of concern. These patients need definite reassessment but not necessarily any intervention.

One major difference between our studies described in this chapter and other reports is that we attempted to individualize the TTS fentanyl dose rate for each patient, whereas the other investigators used the same rate for all patients, usually 100 μg/h. Our approach was based on the premise that it is well known that not all patients have an acceptable level of postoperative pain relief from the same input rate. In fact, there is a five-fold variation in patients' postoperative fentanyl requirements for effective pain control. We attempted to individualize the nominal input rate based upon a number of preoperative psychological assessments and anthropometric parameters that had been shown to correlate with fentanyl demand rates in a previously reported PCA study [8]. However, all our patients required at least one dose of additional pethidine, although the mean amount of supplemental pain relief expressed as a percentage of the placebo group was slightly lower in our studies than the results of Rowbotham et al. [17]. Therefore, the conclusion that modest, if any, gains are achieved by individualizing the dose based on the psychological measures we used is valid. This is not to say that other psychological measures (anxiety, etc.) will prove to be beneficial.

In summary, the TTS fentanyl systems produced fentanyl blood concentrations which should provide a good basis for postoperative analgesia, sometimes after long delay times. Excessive movement of patients after surgery (for example, physiotherapy and mobilization) can produce an increased pain stimulus and an increased requirement for analgesic agents. The results suggest that the TTS fentanyl systems could generate blood fentanyl concentrations to control the "background" level of postoperative pain but any "acute pain episode" or "incident" pain will still require supplementary opioid administration. The range of side effects from the TTS fentanyl systems plus supplementary pethidine are similar to patient-demand intravenous opioid, suggesting that these adverse effects were probably associated with the blood concentrations of the opioids required to provide effective postoperative pain control. Besides the considerable delay before effective analgesic concentrations are achieved, fentanyl blood concentrations remain elevated and decline more slowly than expected once the TTS systems are removed.

References

1. Andrews CJH, Prys-Roberts C (1983) Fentanyl – A Review. Clinics in Anaesthesiol 1: 97–122
2. Austin KL, Stapleton JV, Mather LE (1980) Relationship between blood meperidine concentration and analgesic response: A preliminary report. Anesthestiology 53: 460–466
3. Beck AT, Ward CH, Mendelson M, Monk J, Erbaugh J (1961) An inventory for measuring depression. Arch Gen Psychiatry 4: 53–63
4. Cartwright P, Prys-Roberts C, Gill K, Dye A, Stafford M, Gray A (1983) Ventilatory depression related to plasma fentanyl concentrations during and after anaesthesia in humans. Anesth Analg 62: 966–974
5. Dahlstrom B, Tamsen A, Paalzow L, Hartvig P (1982) Patient controlled analgesic therapy, Part IV: Pharmacokinetics and analgesic plasma concentrations of morphine. Clin Pharmacokinet 7: 266–279
6. Duthie DJR, Rowbotham Dj, Wyld R, Henderson PD, Nimmo WS (1988) Plasma fentanyl concentrations during transdermal delivery of fentanyl to surgical patients. Br J Anaesth 60: 614–618
7. Eysenck HJ, Eysenck SBG (1975) Manual for the Eysenck Personality Questionnaire. Hodder and Stoughton, Kent
8. Gourlay GK, Kowalski, SR, Plummer JL, Cousins MJ, Armstrong PJ (1988) Fentanyl blood concentration – analgesic response relationship in the treatment of postoperative pain. Anesth Analg 67: 329–337
9. Gourlay GK, Kowalski SR, Plummer JL, Cherry DA, Gaukroger P, Cousins MJ (1989) The transdermal administration of fentanyl in the treatment of postoperative pain. Pharmacokinetics and pharmacodynamic effects. Pain 37: 193–202
10. Gourlay GK, Kowalski SR, Plummer JL, Cherry DA, Szekely SM, Mather LE, Owen H, Cousins MJ (1990) The efficacy of transdermal fentanyl in the treatment of postoperative pain: A double blind comparison of fentanyl and placebo systems. Pain 40:21–28
11. Holley FO, van Steennis C (1988) Postoperative analgesia with fentanyl: Pharmacokinetics and pharmacodynamics of constant-rate IV and transdermal delivery. Br J Anaesth 60: 608–613
12. Kowalski SR, Gourlay GK, Cherry DA, McLean CF (1987) A sensitive GLC method for the determination of fentanyl concentrations in blood. J Pharmacol Methods 18: 347–355
13. Lehmann KA (1985) Pharmacokinetics of opioid analgesics. In: Harmer M, Rosen M, Vickers MD (eds) Patient Controlled Analgesia. Blackwell Scientific Publications Oxford, pp 18–29

14. Nimmo WS, Todd JG (1985) Fentanyl by constant rate I.V. infusion for postoperative analgesia. Br J Anaesth 57: 250–254
15. Pilowsky I, Spence ND (1983) Manual for the Illness Behaviour Questionnaire (IBQ), 2nd edn., University of Adelaide, Adelaide
16. Plezia PM, Kramer TH, Linford J, Hameroff SR (1989) Transdermal fentanyl: Pharmacokinetics and preliminary clinical evaluation. Pharmacotherapy 9: 2–9
17. Rowbotham DJ, Wyld R, Peacock JE, Duthie DJR, Nimmo WS (1989) Transdermal fentanyl for the relief of pain after upper abdominal surgery. Br J Anaesth 63: 56–59
18. Rutter PC, Murphy G, Dudley HAF (1980) Morphine: Controlled trial of different methods of administration for postoperative pain relief. Br Med J 1: 12–13
19. Stapleton JV, Austin KL, Mather LE (1979) A pharmacokinetic approach to postoperative pain control: Continuous infusion of pethidine. Anaesth Intens Care 7: 25–32
20. Tamsen A, Hartvig P, Fagerlund C, Dahlstrom B (1982) Patient controlled analgesic therapy, part II: Individual analgesic demand and analgesic plasma concentrations of pethidine in postoperative pain. Clin Pharmacokin 7: 164–175
21. Varvel JR, Shafer SL, Hwang SS, Coen PA, Stanski DR (1989) Absorption characteristics of transdermally administered fentanyl. Anesthesiology 70: 928–934

Clinical Experience

B. von Borman

Introduction

Despite the administration of highly potent analgesics, a large portion of patients complain of pain during the period immediately after surgery. One reason for this is that the conventional methods of administering analgesics do not usually provide a constant level of release [1].

In 1968 Zaffaroni [16] proposed so-called "therapeutic systems" as an alternative to the usual procedures of delivering medication. The object of such systems is to release highly active substances at a constant rate over a certain period of time.

The transdermal application of opioids constitutes a new development. Thus far only clinical studies on their application, particularly during the perioperative period have been performed. In this context only fentanyl has been available in a transdermal therapeutic system (TTS fentanyl). A micropore membrane delivering fentanyl at a constant rate is the underlying construction principle. Release of fentanyl from the transdermal therapeutic system into the skin and thus into the blood stream is characterized by four phases:

1. Saturation of an intracutaneous fentanyl depot
2. Resorption into the blood stream to attain a steady state concentration (until removal of system)
3. Continued resorption of fentanyl after removing the system, as the intracutaneous fentanyl depot is emptied
4. Pure elimination phase, induced by fentanyl metabolism

In individual cases the fentanyl concentration may continue to increase after the patch is removed, depending on the skin texture, hemodynamic conditions, and local blood circulation. Pharmacokinetic effects of transdermal fentanyl may explain advantages, disadvantages and risks of this mode of pain treatment.

Methods and Results of Recent Studies

All investigations performed to date focus on the following parameters:
- Analgetic effect by pain score or observing nurses' statement
- Analgetic effect by demand of supplemental opioid therapy
- Blood (serum) concentrations of fentanyl
- Handling
- Acceptance
- Side effects
  - Erythema (blistering)
  - Pruritus
  - Nausea
  - Vomiting
  - Urinary retention
  - Respiratory depression

The investigations were performed on patients with different surgical procedures such as lower and upper abdominal surgery, minor and major orthopedic surgery (performed under general anesthesia as well as epidural analgesia), spinal analgesia, and blockade of plexus axillaris [2–5, 7–15].

Handling and Acceptance

No problems in handling the TTS fentanyl patch have been reported. Some patients had local erythema after removal of the system. Caplan et al. [4] reported that about 59% of patients of the active group (verum), and 35% of the placebo group, showed erythema after patch removal. By 24 h, all topical changes had disappeared except for one patient of the active group who had a blistered area. This lesion resolved without sequelae.

Acceptance of the method by the patients was about 100% in all studies. There were no reports of any patient refusing TTS fentanyl treatment.

Pain Control

Overall satisfaction with pain control was expressed by 60%–85% of patients with verum application; even up to 45% of patients with placebo were likewise satisfied [2, 5, 12, 14]. Studies with double blind, placebo-controlled, randomized design demonstrated that spontaneous remarks about an agreeable "constant" quality of pain control were made only by patients with active transdermal systems [3, 4, 9–11, 14].

During the period in which the systems were in place (typically 24 h), and during the first 12-h period after removal, patients using the active system had significantly lower visual analogue scores than patients with placebo.

Patients using the active system required significantly less supplemental narcotic than patients using the placebo system (Fig. 1). These findings are in accordance with those from several other groups.

Though there is no linear correlation between particular pain control and the serum level of narcotics in an individual, a relationship between blood opioid concentration and postoperative pain relief has been established [1, 6]. As demonstrated in Fig. 2, most patients with pain score values = 0 (no pain) had fentanyl levels ranging from 0.70 to 1.3 ng/ml [3].

Several communications have also shown that the effect of TTS fentanyl systems is slow: there is a delay time of 3–37 h before fentanyl blood concentrations exceed the previously determined values of minimal effective concentration (MEC) [2, 3, 7–9, 15]. As serum fentanyl levels are quite low for a number of hours after placement of the transdermal system, it would be reasonable to apply it prior to surgery and provide analgesia by parenterally administered opioids for the first several hours after system application. Therefore, several groups have applied a bolus of fentanyl ranging from 0.1 to 0.925 mg (including continuous i.v. infusion) at induction of anesthesia [2, 7, 8, 10, 12, 14, 15].

The slow decline in serum fentanyl levels offers a potential advantage in that the transition to other forms of pain management may occur without an abrupt loss of analgesia. However, if prompt and complete termination of narcotic effect is desired, serial injections or continuous infusion of a narcotic antagonist may be required until the skin depot is sufficiently depleted [4, 5].

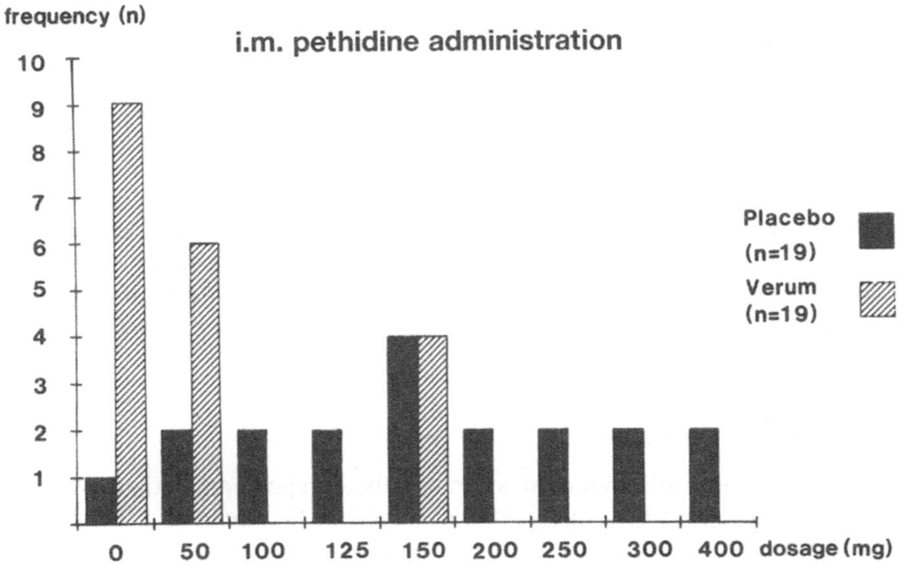

Fig. 1. Additive pain therapy in patients with F-TTS (verum, placebo resp.). It is demonstrated how much pethidine in total was required by how many of the patients (frequency)

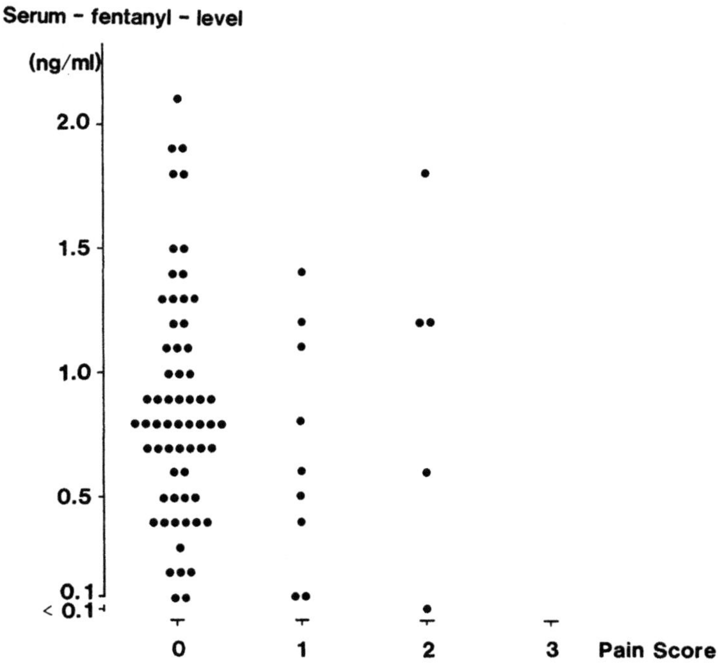

Fig. 2. Relationship between pain score and fentanyl blood-level in patients with F-TTS (verum)

Side Effects

Several placebo-controlled studies demonstrated side effects such as nausea, vomiting, urinary retention, and pruritus independently of the mode of treatment (transdermal plus i v/i m opioid vs i v/i m opioid alone).

In contrast to others, Caplan and coworkers [4] reported a statistically significant difference for vomiting which was less pronounced in patients with placebo (73% and 30% respectively). Latasch and coworkers, however, found no vomiting, no urinary retention and no skin reactions caused by the patches, whereas nine patients with TTS fentanyl but none with placebo complained about itching [11].

Respiratory Depression

Single cases of respiratory depression have been reported. Ventilatory rate in two patients with TTS fentanyl 100, observed by Duthie et al. [7] decreased to less than eight breaths/min during sleep. Plasma fentanyl levels at these times were 2.8 and 2.9 ng/ml. Both patients had supplementary morphine (20 mg and 10 mg, respectively). In our own study a woman with a severe respiratory depression was treated with TTS fentanyl 75 (Fig. 3). After the

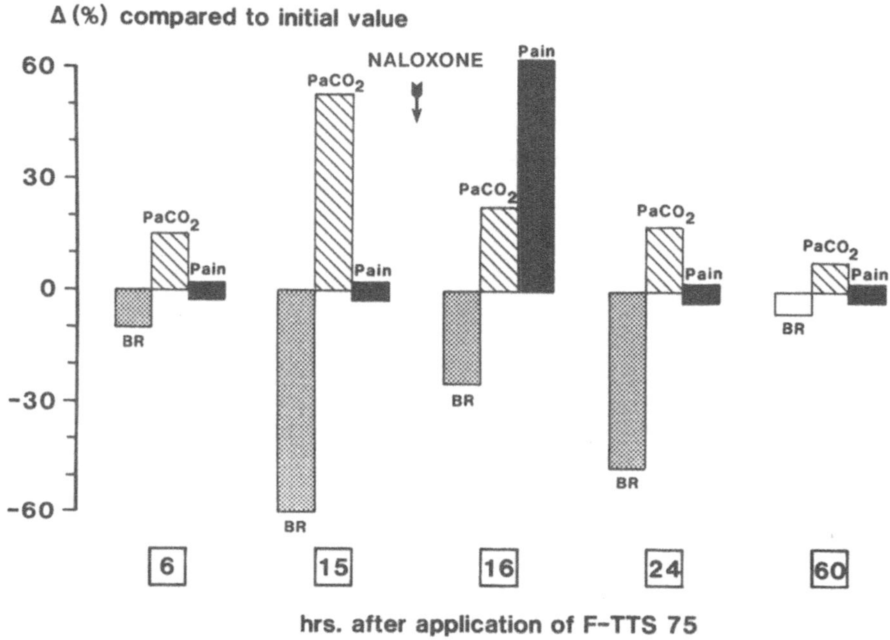

Fig. 3. Respiratory data in a patient with F-TTS and severe respiratory depression. BR = breathing rate

system had been applied for 15 h the respiratory rate dropped to six breaths/min and the carbon dioxide tension increased to 59 mmHg. The patient became drowsy and did not complain of pain. After administering naloxone iv the respiratory function improved markedly and the patient suffered from intensive pain. Fentanyl serum levels increased continuously, to a maximum of 3.2 ng/ml (Fig. 4), even after removal of the patch (24th hour). Although respiratory depression cannot generally be predicted on the basis of opioid concentration in the blood [6], the connection in this case seems to be significant.

The recent literature seems to provide no correlation between specific methods or circumstances and respiratory depression: respiratory depression has not been correlated with the mode of anesthesia (general, spinal, epidural plus general, interscalene block), the type of surgery (abdominal or orthopedic, minor or major), the quantity of a given loading dose (0.1–1.0 mg fentanyl, commonly applied prior to operation), the delivery rate (25–125 μg/h), or the narcotic used for supplementary analgesia (morphine, piritramide, pethidine) [7, 8, 10, 11]. Therefore, prediction of respiratory depression may be impossible.

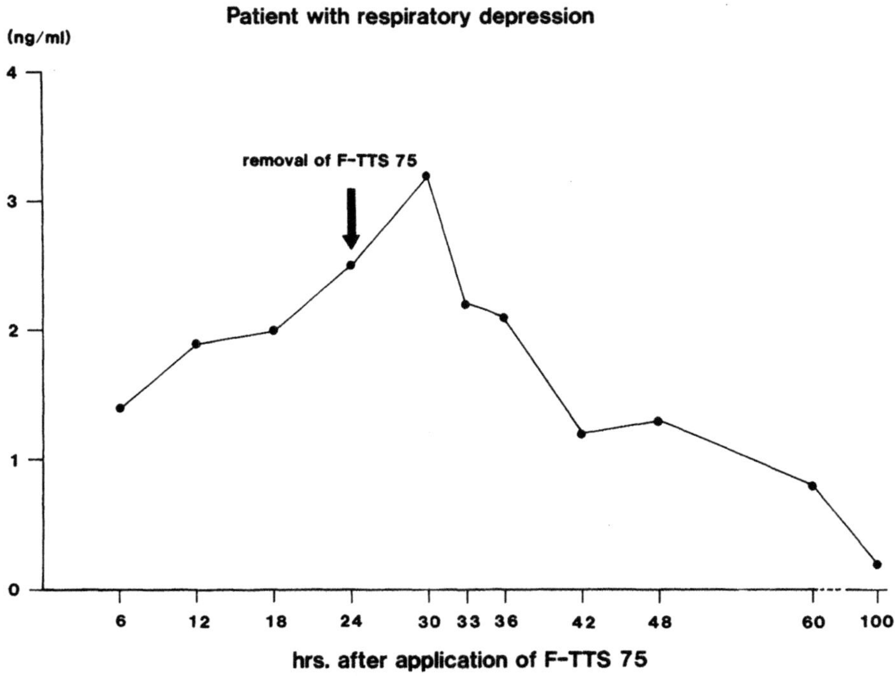

Fig. 4. Fentanyl blood-levels of the patient demonstrated in Fig. 3

Conclusions

The delivery of an opioid by the transdermal route may be useful in the treatment of pain after surgery. Most authors demonstrated a high quality of pain control using TTS fentanyl in surgical patients. One advantage of TTS fentanyl is the ability to maintain a relatively constant drug concentration for a prolonged period of time by avoiding invasive techniques. On the other hand, the opiate loading dose has to be given prior to surgery as verum fentanyl levels are quite low for a number of hours after replacement of transdermal systems [15]. Delay time before onset of adequate analgesia may be 3 to 37 (!) hours [8, 9].

Severe respiratory depression is rare but may occur even without additional narcotics, as demonstrated by our own group (Figs. 3, 4) [3]. This variability necessitates the same monitoring for opioid side effects when using this transdermal fentanyl system as is needed when using parenteral routes with constant rate application independent of individual patients' needs. It should be borne in mind that some patients, albeit few, require no analgesia after surgery.

TTS fentanyl is a system capable of releasing fentanyl into systemic circulation via the unbroken skin. The drug is stored in a skin depot resulting in continuous drug delivery into the blood even after removal of the patch.

Effects, side effects, and problems of transdermal opioid treatment are nearly identical to those known for any form of narcotic therapy.

Pain therapy in acute (postoperative) pain should be regulated by patients' demand provided by intravenous application in the form of so-called patient-controlled analgesia. Although the dosage of TTS fentanyl can be customized it is not possible to achieve the same fine degree of titration that is offered by iv infusion.

Uncontrollable delay, unpredictable development of respiratory depression even after removal of the patch (skin depot!), and the impossibility of time-related individual dosage exclude the transdermal fentanyl system from routine administration in postoperative patients.

References

1. Austin KL, Stapleton JV, Mather LE (1980) Relationship between blood meperidine concentration and analgesic response. Anesthesiology 53: 460
2. Bell SD, Goldberg ME, Larijani GE, Marr AT, Rudloff G (1989) Evaluation of transdermal fentanyl for multi-day analgesia in postoperative patients. Anesth Analg 68: S22
3. v. Bormann B, Ratthey K, Schwetlick G, Schneider Ch, Müller H, Hempelmann G (1988) Postoperative Schmerztherapie durch transdermales Fentanyl. Anästh Intensivther Notfallmed 23: 3
4. Caplan RA, Ready LB, Oden RV, Matsen III FA, Nessly ML, Olsson GL (1989) Transdermal fentanyl for postoperative pain management. JAMA 261: 1036
5. Caplan RA, Southam M (1990) Transdermal drug delivery and its application to pain control. Adv in Pain Res Ther 14: 233
6. Cartwright P, Prys-Roberts C, Gill K, Dye A, Stafford M, Gray A (1983) Ventilatory depression related to plasma fentanyl concentrations during and after anesthesia in humans. Anesth Analg 62: 966
7. Duthie DJR, Rowbotham DJ, Wyld R, Henderson PD, Nimmo WS (1988) Plasma fentanyl concentrations during transdermal delivery of fentanyl to surgical patients. Br J Anaesth 60:614
8. Gourlay GK, Kowalski StR, Plummer JL, Cherry DA, Gaukroger Ph, Cousins MJ (1989) The transdermal administration of fentanyl in the treatment of postoperative pain: pharmacokinetics and pharmacodynamic effects. Pain 37: 193
9. Gourlay GK, Kowalski StR, Plummer JL, Cherry DA, Szekely SM, Mather LE, Owen H, Cousins MJ (1990) The efficacy of transdermal fentanyl in the treatment of postoperative pain: a double-blind comparison of fentanyl and placebo system. Pain 40: 21
10. Holley FO, van Steenis C (1988) Postoperative analgesia with fentanyl: pharmacokinetics and pharmacodynamics of constant-rate i.v. and transdermal delivery. Br J Anaesth 60: 608
11. Latasch, L, Lüders S (1989) Transdermal fentanyl against postoperative pain. Acta Anaesth Belg 40: 113
12. Mc Leskey, Mac Rae J (1990) Transdermal fentanyl for postoperative pain following lower abdominal surgery. Anesth Analg 70:S264
13. Plezia PM, Linford J, Kramer TH, Iacono RP, Hameroff SR (1986) Transdermal therapeutic system (fentanyl) for postoperative pain: An efficacy, toxicity, and pharmacokinetic trial. Anesthesiology 65: A210

14. Rowbotham DJ, Wyld R, Peacock JE, Duthie DJR (1989) Transdermal fentanyl for the relief of pain after upper abdominal surgery. Br J Anaesth 63: 56
15. Varvel JR, Shafer SL, Hwang SS, Coen PA, Stanski DR (1989) Absorption characteristics of transdermally administered fentanyl. Anesthesiology 70: 928
16. Zaffaroni A (1970) Towards a new concept in drug administration. Pharm J 205: 400

Respiratory Safety

L. LATASCH and R. CHRIST

Introduction

Opioid-induced respiratory depression is one effect which, in addition to the abuse potential of μ-agonist opioids, limits the applicability of this group of pharmacological agents. In the presence of acute or chronic pain, addiction is very seldom seen.

While psychic and physical dependence develop after repeated injection of an opioid, respiratory depression is an acute effect occurring immediately after the injection. The various opioids differ in their ability to induce respiratory depression. In general, the respiratory depressant potential mirrors the analgetic potency of an opioid in a directly proportional manner.

Fentanyl, the active ingredient of TTS fentanyl, is a classic μ-agonist analgesic. Like most opioids, it induces a central respiratory depression, mainly by reducing the sensitivity of the "respiratory center" towards CO_2 [2, 6]. This reduction of sensitivity in turn triggers a rightward shift in the CO_2 response curve and is also accompanied by a reduction of arterial O_2-saturation.

Following the intravenous injection of a centrally acting opioid, the following pattern can be observed:
- *Phase 1,* period in which respiratory rate decreases (bradypnea).
- *Phase 2,* phase in which respiration requires external stimulation (acoustically, nociceptively or optically) [7]. This phase is relatively short-lived, barely detectable, and quickly followed by Phase 3.
- *Phase 3,* where respiration requires active efforts by the patient, triggered through verbal command by the physician [1, 13].

If the administered amount of the opioid is large enough, apnea is the final result.

Although both respiratory depression and the analgesic properties of opioids are dose-related, respiratory depression can occur at subanalgesic doses of these agents. There is no direct correlation of opioid plasma levels and respiratory depression, although some authors report that the plasma level producing clinically relevant respiratory depression for fentanyl may be as low as 3 ng/ml [8]. Lehmann and coauthors could not detect clinically relevant respiratory depression even at peak plasma levels of 6.8 ng fentanyl/ml plasma, even though in another study [12] the authors state that after the application of fentanyl, the recovery period of the respiratory center was clearly prolonged (after fentanyl) and that (even after 60 min) the sensitivity of the respiratory center for CO_2 was reduced by 35% as compared to pre-experimental data.

Reduction of Vigilance

A blockade of the nociceptive afference by fentanyl simultaneously induces a disruption of the polysynaptic conduction in the activating reticular system leading to the cortex, thereby reducing vigilance. This hypnotic effect characterizes many opioids. Combinations with other CNS depressants (e.g., barbiturates, benzodiazepines, or neuroleptics) intensify and prolong the respiratory depressant effects by further reducing vigilance. In addition, other factors such as preexisting respiratory disease, old age, hypoproteinemia, hypothermia, or drug interaction (β-blockers, antidepressants, cytostatics, etc.) may lead to a potentiation of the opioid effects on respiration.

In a recent study by the authors, carried out with E. Freye, Düsseldorf, we applied a dose of 21 μg/kg sufentanil to waking dogs after blocking the μ-receptor.

Breathing ambient air, 5 min after the application of sufentanil, either a μ- or δ-antagonist was given to reverse respiratory depression. In order to evaluate the relationship between the state of vigilance, as reflected in the various EEG power bands, and the change in arterial blood gases, correlation equations were computed. Figure 1 shows a close *linear* correlation ($r = 0.99$) between values in the delta-band plotted against the $PaCO_2$ values following different medications. However, computation of linear correlation of changes in the PaO_2 and the power in the delta- as well as the beta domain is not ideal ($r = 0.74$). When computing the *logarithmic* correlation of PaO_2 against power in the beta band following administration of different antagonists, the correlation coefficient is much higher ($r = 0.975$) (Fig. 2). This finding seems to indicate that PaO_2 and $PaCO_2$ are affected independently of each other by opioids, while both regulate the rhythmic discharge of respiratory neurons in the reticular system. Vigilance seems to be the key element in the regulation of respiration.

Clinical Data

In a double blind study performed in 1988 [10], 60 patients (ASA class I–II) undergoing knee arthrotomy received a transdermal drug delivery system containing either fentanyl, TTS fentanyl, or placebo (nominal delivery rate 75 μg/h). As in other studies, the system remained in place for 24 h. The aim of

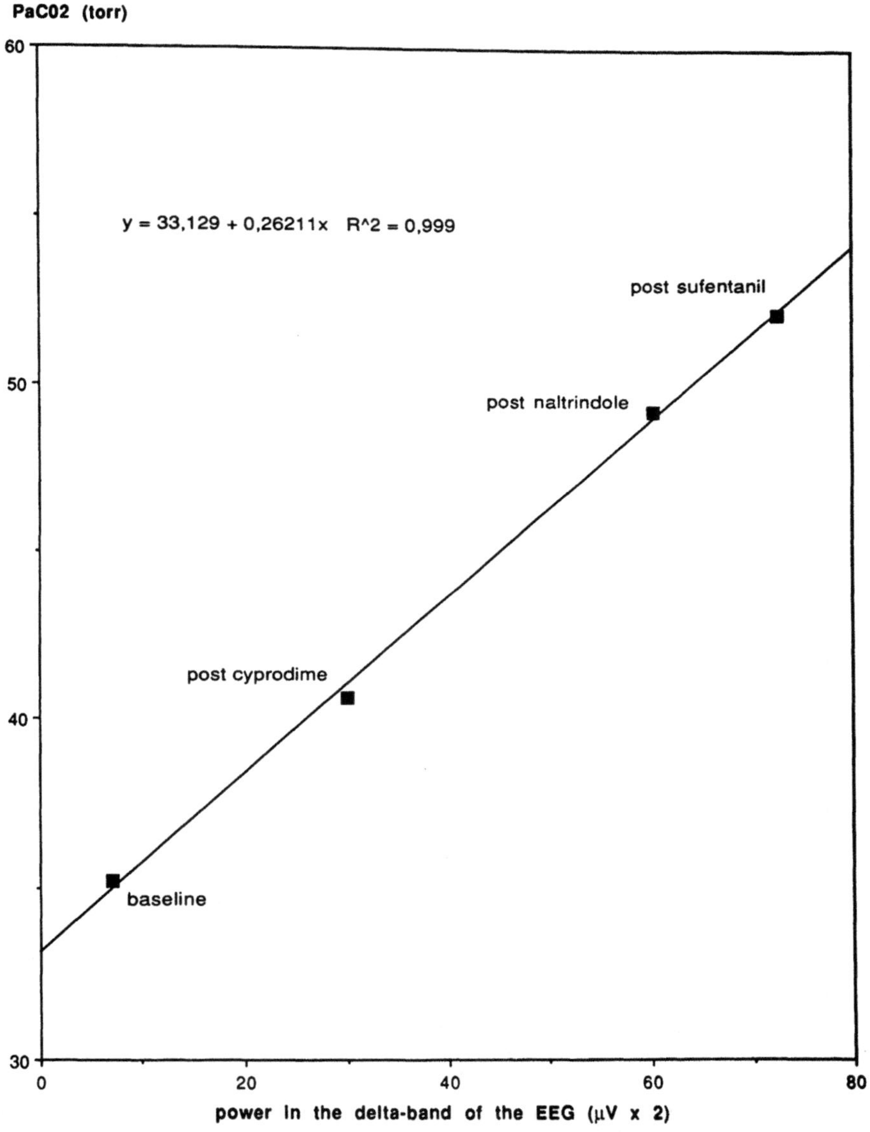

Fig. 1. Linear correlation between the power in the delta-band of the EEG and the corresponding $PaCO_2$ values. The high correlation coefficient suggests a close interaction between deactivation of cortical activity and hypercapnia

our study was to evaluate the effects of TTS fentanyl on respiration, with the attempt to define a standard pattern of parameters for respiratory function.

For the operation, spinal anesthesia (bupivacaine and adrenaline) lasting approximately 3.7 h was performed. The transdermal system was applied

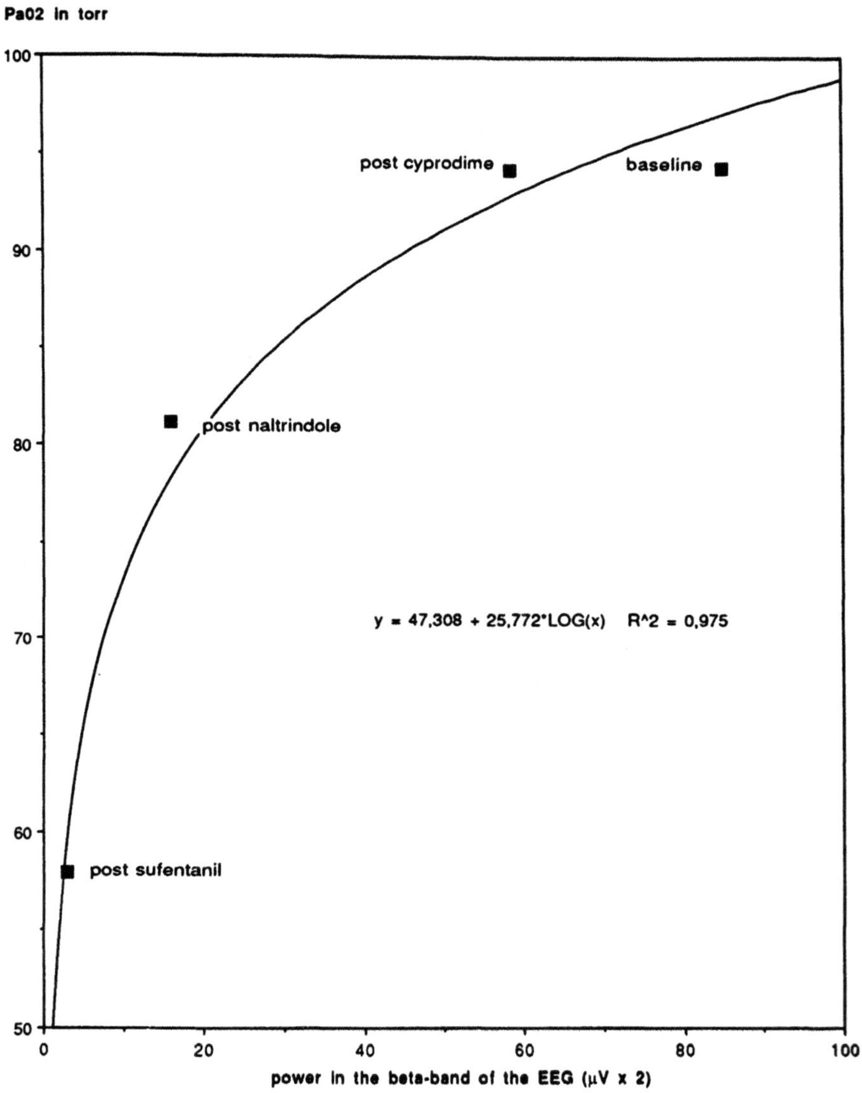

Fig. 2. Computation of logarithmic correlation between power in the beta-band of the EEG and the corresponding PaO_2 values. The data suggests that the increase in vigilance results in a sufficient respiratory drive which reverses hypoxemia

immediately prior to surgery. After the operation, piritramide (7.5 mg i.m.) was allowed as escape analgesia. If the patient still complained about pain after receiving the first dose of piritramide, the 7.5 mg could be doubled after 1 h. While the total amount of piritramide was not restricted, the amount of piritramide/h was limited.

Respiratory minute volume, tidal volume, forced expiratory volume and forced expiratory vital capacity were measured 3, 6, 10 and 24 h after system application. The definition of respiratory depression was based upon laboratory data as well as the overall clinical picture. For clinical evaluation the following parameters were taken into account:

1. Breaths/min
2. Consciousness (arousable or unarousable)
3. Respiratory minute volume and forced expiratory volume
4. Possible cyanosis

Physiological standards for PO_2 were assumed as 70–100 mmHg (9.31–13.3 kPa), and, for PCO_2, 36–45 mmHg (4.78–5.98 kPa).

All these data were compared with those taken prior to surgery, so that even if laboratory data were to indicate incipient respiratory depression, evaluation of "all" data could avoid possible medical therapy.

Results

Apart from patient 1, the values of PO_2 (Fig. 3), PCO_2 (Fig. 4), respiratory minute volume (Fig. 5), tidal volume, forced expiratory volume, and forced expiratory vital capacity did not differ between the patients of both groups (fentanyl vs placebo), even when piritramide was added.

Six hours after application of the transdermal system, patient 1 had a PCO_2 of 51 mmHg (6.78 Pa) and a PO_2 of 65 mmHg (8.65 Pa) (Fig. 6). He showed

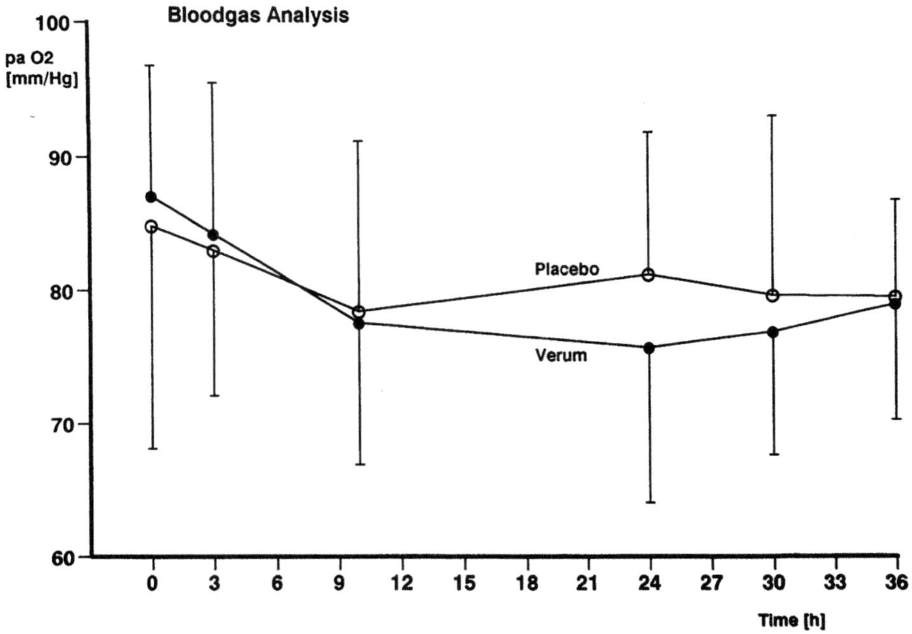

Fig. 3. Comparison of PaO_2 between the verum (fentanyl) and the placebo group (Mean values ± SD)

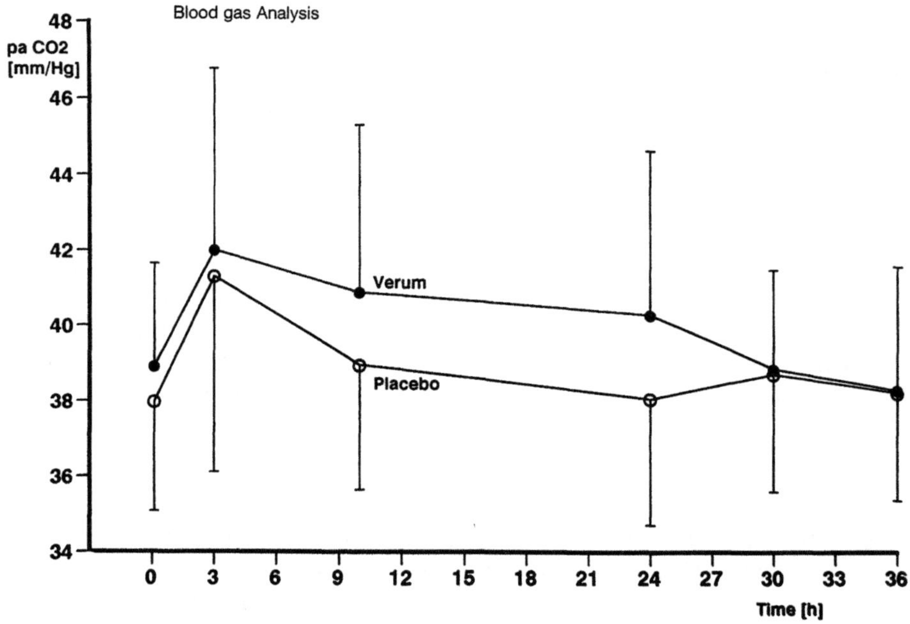

Fig. 4. Comparison of $PaCO_2$ between the verum (fentanyl) and the placebo group (Mean values ± SD)

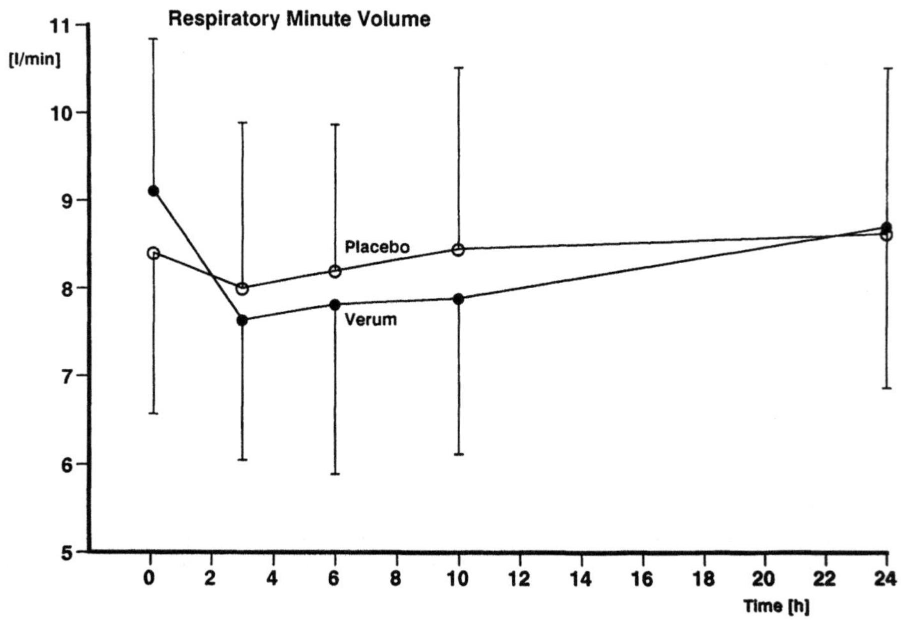

Fig. 5. Comparison of respiratory parameters (respiratory minute volume) of the fentanyl (verum) and placebo group (Mean values ± SD)

moderate sedation, no peripheral cyanosis, an average of more than 9 breaths/min, and was never unarousable. His serum level of fentanyl was nearly three times higher than the average level of the other patients. Comparing the high serum levels of patient 1 with those of other patients, we found a direct correlation between body weight, patch size, and fentanyl serum levels.

Body weight of patient 1 was 50 kg, the lowest allowed in this study. Patients weighing between 50 and 60 kg were also compared, and the above-mentioned positive correlation was found here as well.

It is very difficult to compare our results with those obtained in other studies done with TTS fentanyl in regard to respiratory safety, because there are no "standard procedures" for monitoring and evaluation. Some studies use the measurement of respiratory rate (b.p.m.) as the only parameter for respiratory function [3–5]. As Holley and van Steennis [9] found, ventilatory rate is not helpful in detecting hypercapnia: the rate in patients with $PaCO_2 >$ 6.7 kPa (50 mmHg) ranged from 7 to 22 breaths/min. In patients with ventilatory rates of 10 or less, they found $PaCO_2$ values ranging from 3.3 (25 mmHg) to 7.1 kPa (54 mmHg).

In the course of their studies other authors have given the patients additional oxygen, as Holley did for a period of 12 h postoperatively because of PaO_2 values < 9.3 kPa (70 mmHg), thereby altering the true blood gas measurements.

In evaluating the complex situation of respiratory depression ventilatory rate does not seem adequate as a safety measure in clinical practice. TTS fentanyl causes sedation, thereby reducing vigilance.

Summary and Conclusion

Vigilance seems to be the factor which transforms a nonrelevant "respiratory depression" into a clinically relevant one demanding therapeutic intervention. Therefore, none of the patients treated with TTS fentanyl should receive sleeping medication or any additional medication causing extra sedation during the period when wearing the transdermal system. Moreover, we see no necessity to give supplemental oxygen after application of the transdermal system. In our opinion, there should be a limitation by body weight for the different sizes of the patches (< 60 kg: 50 µg/h, 60–90 kg: 75 µg/h, and > 90 kg: 100 µg/h. If additional safety measurements are wanted, a pulse oximeter should be used.

If all these "precautions" are taken, no clinically relevant respiratory depression should occur, and TTS fentanyl would be considered safe and effective for the treatment of postoperative pain.

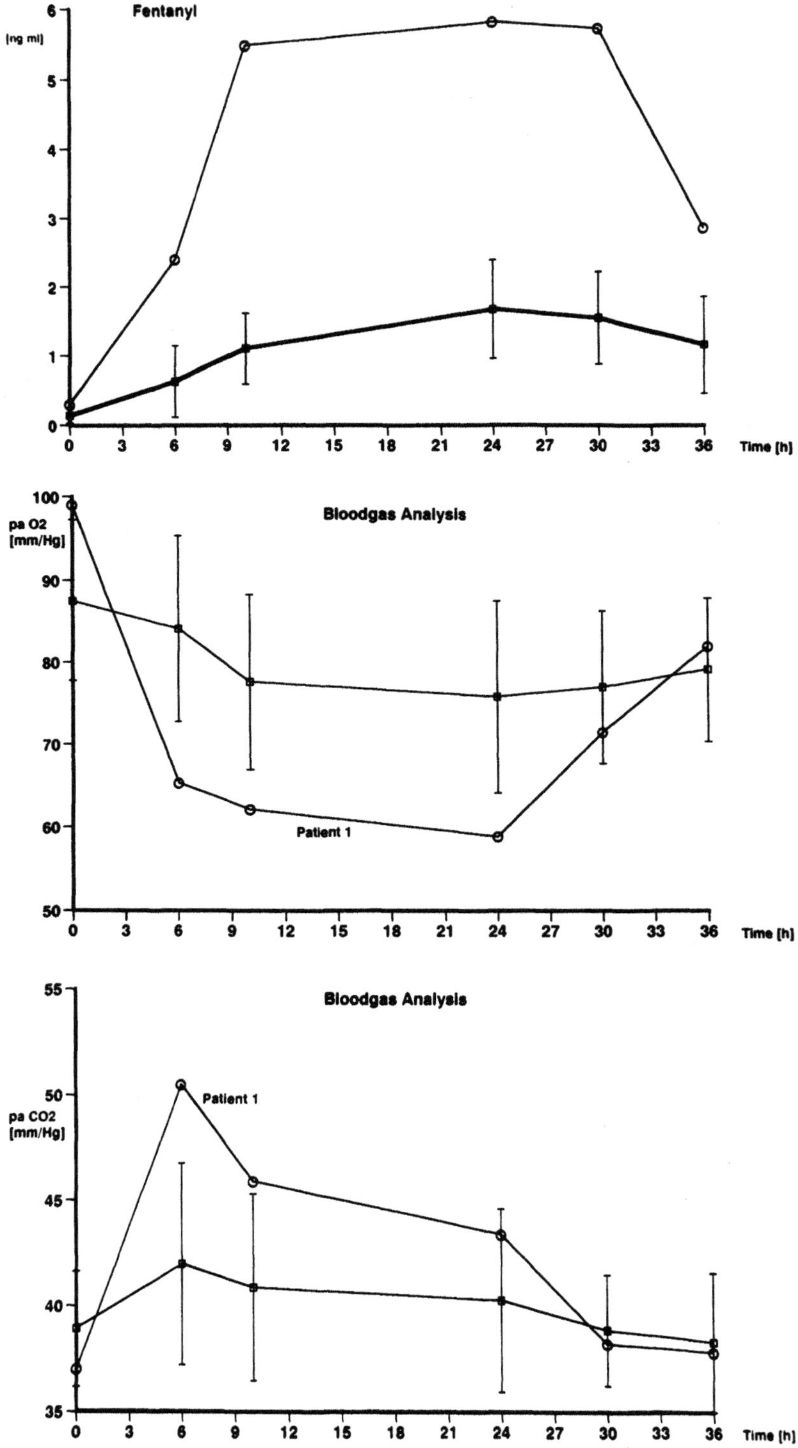
Fentanyl
[ng ml]
6
5
4
3
2
1
0
0 3 6 9 12 15 18 21 24 27 30 33 36
Time [h]
Bloodgas Analysis
pa O2
[mm/Hg]
100
90
80
70
60
50
Patient 1
0 3 6 9 12 15 18 21 24 27 30 33 36
Time [h]
Bloodgas Analysis
pa CO2
[mm/Hg]
55
50
45
40
35
Patient 1
0 3 6 9 12 15 18 21 24 27 30 33 36
Time [h]

References

1. Bedford RF, Wollmann H (1975) Postoperative respiratory effects of morphine and halothane anesthesia: a study in patients undergoing cardiac surgery. Anesthesiology 43: 1
2. Bellville JW, Seed JC (1960) The effect of drugs on the respiratory response to carbon dioxide. Anesthesiology 21: 727
3. Caplan RA, Ready B, Oden RV, Matsen FA, Nessly ML, Olsson GK (1989) Transdermal fentanyl for postoperative pain treatment. JAMA 261: 1036
4. Duthie DJR, McLaren AD, Nimmo WS (1986) Pharmacokinetics of fentanyl during constant rate i.v. infusion for the relief of pain after surgery. Br J Anesth 58: 950
5. Duthie DJR, Rowbotham DJ, Wyld R, Henderson PD, Nimmo WS (1988) Plasma fentanyl concentrations during transdermal delivery of fentanyl to surgical patients. Br J Anaesth 60: 614
6. Eisenmann AJ, Martin WR (1961) Effect of morphine and nalorphine on serum CO_2, serum pH and respiratory rate in the decerebrate rat. Fed Proc 20: 310
7. Eckenhoff JE, Oechs R (1960) The effects of narcotics and antagonists on respiration and circulation in man. Clin Pharm Therapeut 1: 483
8. Hill HF (1990) The pharmacology of transdermal fentanyl. Abstract: New opioid techniques in pain treatment. VI World Congress on Pain, Adelaide, 1–6 April 1990
9. Holley FO, van Steennis C (1988) Postoperative analgesia with fentanyl: pharmacokinetics and pharmacodynamics of constant-rate i.v. and transdermal delivery. Br J Anaesth 60: 608
10. Latasch L, Lüders S (1989) Transdermal Fentanyl against postoperative pain. Acta Anaesth Belg 40. 113
11. Lehmann KA, Neubauer ML, Mainka F, Daub D (1982) CO_2-Antwort nach Fentanyl und Alfetanil. Anaesthesist 31: 487
12. Lehmann KA, Freier J, Daub D (1982) Fentanyl-Pharmakokinetik und postoperative Atemdepression. Anaesthesist 31: 111
13. Stanley TH, Philbin DM, Coggins CH (1979) Fentanyl-oxygen anaesthesia for coronary artery surgery: cardiovascular and antidiuretic hormone responses. Can Anaesth Soc J 26: 168

◀ **Fig. 6.** Comparison of the fentanyl serum levels *(upper part)* and blood gas values (PaO_2 and $PaCO_2$) between patient 1 and all other patients receiving TTS fentanyl (Mean values ± SD)

TTS Fentanyl in Combination with Patient-Controlled Analgesia

C. EINNOLF, H. J. EBERLEIN, and K. A. LEHMANN

Introduction

Patient-controlled analgesia (PCA) has proved to be a highly effective method of acute pain management which has been well accepted by patients. Given that postoperative analgesic consumption reflects the intensity of postoperative pain, the concept of therapeutic intravenous on-demand analgesia or PCA can be used as a method to quantify postoperative pain [18]. Assuming that the amount of fentanyl required during PCA reflects the quality of pain relief provided by simultaneously performed pain therapy, PCA can be used to quantify the analgesic effect of TTS fentanyl.

The aim of the randomized, double blind study reported in this chapter was to determine the efficacy of TTS fentanyl for postoperative pain relief after major urological operations performed under standardized anesthesia. During PCA all patients, even those with placebo TTS, had the possibility of self-administering intravenous fentanyl whenever they experienced recurring pain. Concerning pain management they were completely independent of medical staff.

Patients and Methods

After the Ethics Committee's approval and after informed written consent had been given, 50 patients scheduled for major elective urological surgery (17 women and 33 men aged 23 to 75, ASA classification I–III) were randomly assigned to two groups (Table 1). Group 1 received a fentanyl transdermal system (TTS) and group 2 a placebo. The TTS was applied to a hair-free area of the upper thorax 8 h before induction of anesthesia. The delivery rate of the transdermal system containing fentanyl was 75 μg/h (Table 2).

All patients were premedicated with midazolam intramuscularly. Anesthesia was induced with thiopentone and maintained with isoflurane, fentanyl, nitrous oxide in oxygen, and vecuronium. A single intravenous fentanyl dose (0.1 mg) was injected immediately prior to skin incision. Further fentanyl injections (0.05–0.1 mg) were given during anesthesia when clinical signs of pain were noticed, such as 20% increases in blood pressure and heart rate,

Table 1. Details of patients

Total number	50 (17 women, 33 men)
Age	23–75 years
ASA classification	I–III
Type of urological surgery	nephrectomy, cystectomy, transvesical prostatectomy, nephro- and ureterolithotomy, removal of paraaortic lymphatic nodes
Group I	Verum-TTS (n = 25)
Group II	Placebo-TTS (n = 25)

Table 2. Methods

Application of the test system 8 h before anesthesia
Standardized anesthesia (incl. one 100 μg fentanyl i.v. bolus)
PCA (18 ± 3 h) with fentanyl: bolus 34 μg, max. 408 μg/h;
Hourly documentation of blood pressure, heart rate, respiratory rate, pain intensity (VAS 0–100), and side effects
Arterial blood gas analyses
Postoperative interview

lacrimation, or sweating. Ninety min prior to extubation fentanyl was no longer applied.

As soon as the patients were fully orientated in the recovery room, they were connected to a PCA pump (Prominject, Pharmacia, [27]) and were encouraged to self-administer fentanyl doses set at 34 μg whenever they experienced recurring pain. The pump refractory time was 5 min, thus limiting the hourly maximum dose to 0.4 mg intravenously. PCA was maintained until the following morning.

To prevent nausea and vomiting, an intravenous dose of 1 mg droperidol was administered at the beginning of PCA. This dose was repeated whenever necessary.

Blood pressure, heart rate, respiratory rate, pain intensity (using a visual analogue scale, VAS, 0–100), and side effects were documented hourly during the first 10 postoperative hours. All valid demands were automatically recorded along with the exact time of day.

Arterial blood gas analyses were performed at the beginning of PCA and afterwards if and when clinically indicated. Exclusion criteria for the study were

a) respiratory rates of less than 8 breaths/min for a period of more than 5 min,
b) a $PaCO_2$ of more than 55 mmHg, and
c) insufficient pain relief.

No patient had to be excluded.

Table 3. Retrospective verbal pain score

0	No pain at all
1	Sometimes moderate pain
2	Moderate pain at times
3	Severe pain at times
4	Continuous moderate pain, severe at times
5	Discontinuation due to insufficient analgesia

The TTS was removed 24 h after application. Local skin reactions were registered immediately and 1, 6, and 24 h after TTS removal.

On postoperative day 4 patients were interviewed using a standard protocol to evaluate their acceptance of pain relief. The protocol consisted of a retrospective verbal pain score (Table 3) and a VAS.

The SPSS program was used for the statistical analysis including arithmetic means, standard deviations and ranges. The two groups were compared using the Student's *t* test for unpaired values, the Mann-Whitney U-test for independent values, and the chi-square test. *P* values of less than 0.05 were considered statistically significant.

Results

The two groups were similar with regard to age, sex, weight, height, smoking habits, and preoperative consumption of analgesics and alcohol.

The duration of anesthesia did not differ between the two groups. TTS fentanyl proved to be effective during anesthesia since significantly less fentanyl was given intravenously in the verum group (Table 4).

During PCA, individual fentanyl supplementation was highly variable in both groups. Figure 1 represents 25 patients from the TTS fentanyl group. Each line represents one patient, showing cumulative dose-time plots with steps marking the valid demands.

Figure 2 displays the time course of the mean cumulative PCA fentanyl dose of the two groups. The asterisks represent the TTS fentanyl group and the open symbols represent the TTS placebo group.

The duration of PCA was similar in both groups (Table 5). Mean cumulative intravenous fentanyl consumption was significantly less in the verum group, the TTS fentanyl group having a mean total dose of 0.66 mg vs

Table 4. Anaesthesiological data (mean ± SD)

Parameters	TTS fentanyl	TTS placebo	Significance
Duration of anesthesia (min)	255.2 ± 113.9	227.1 ± 77.5	n.s.
Intraoperative fentanyl (ng/kg/min)	7.4 ± 3.3	10.8 ± 3.5	$p = 0.001$

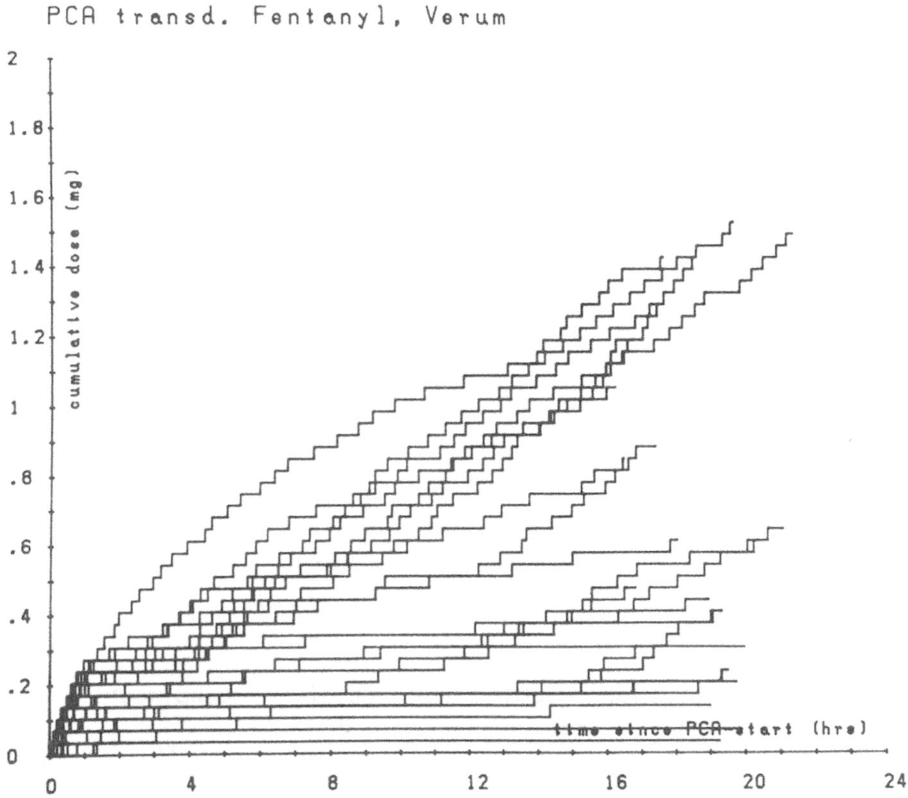

Fig. 1. Individual cumulative dose-time plots of the 25 patients in the TTS fentanyl group. Each step indicates a valid demand; a similar variability was observed with patients of the TTS placebo group (not shown)

1.13 mg for the TTS placebo group. The calculated mean doses of fentanyl demanded were 35.8 and 68.7 μg/h respectively.

Actual VAS pain scores differed significantly between the groups from the third to the ninth hour after PCA was initiated (Fig. 3). This difference between the two groups could not be reproduced with retrospective pain scoring (Table 6).

Table 5. Patient-controlled analgesia – results

Parameters	TTS fentanyl	TTS placebo	Significance
Duration of PCA (h)	18.6 ± 1.4	17.7 ± 4.0	n.s.
PCA fentanyl i.v. application			
– cumulative dose (mg)	0.66 ± 0.49	1.13 ± 0.46	$p = 0.001$
– hourly dosage (μg/h)	35.8 ± 27.1	68.7 ± 32.2	$p < 0.001$

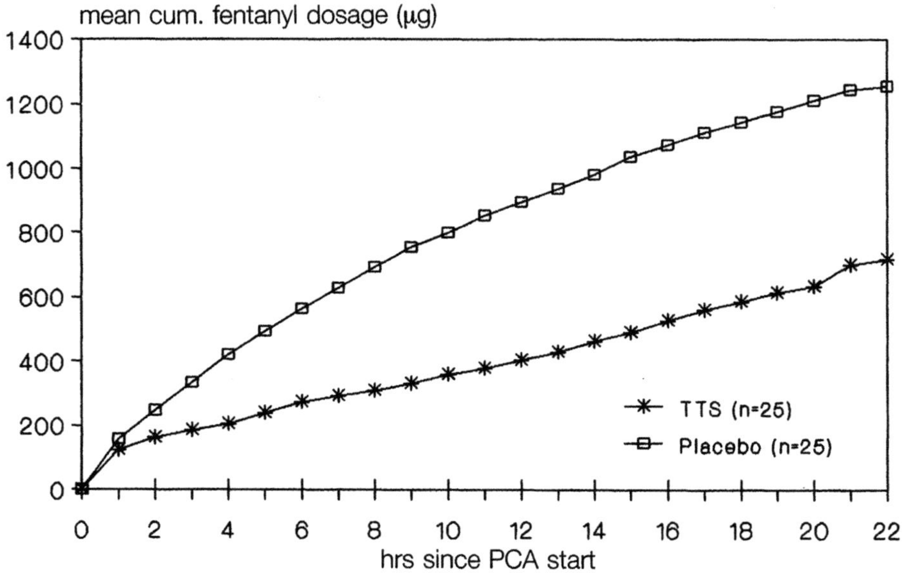

Fig. 2. Mean cumulative PCA fentanyl dosages in the subgroups

There was no statistically significant difference between the groups as far as the hemodynamic parameters were concerned.

Mean respiratory rates were lower in the verum group. The difference, although clinically irrelevant, was statistically significant during a period 8–10

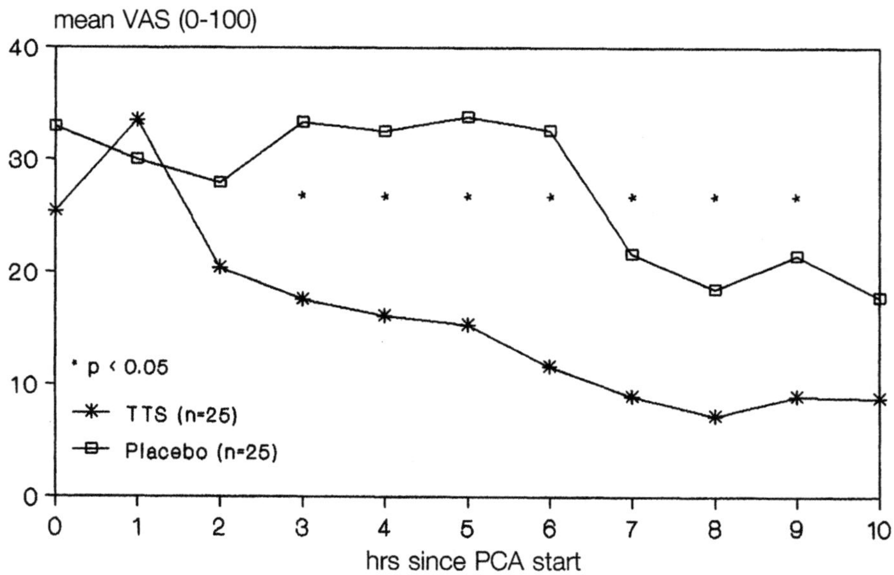

Fig. 3. Mean pain scores during PCA

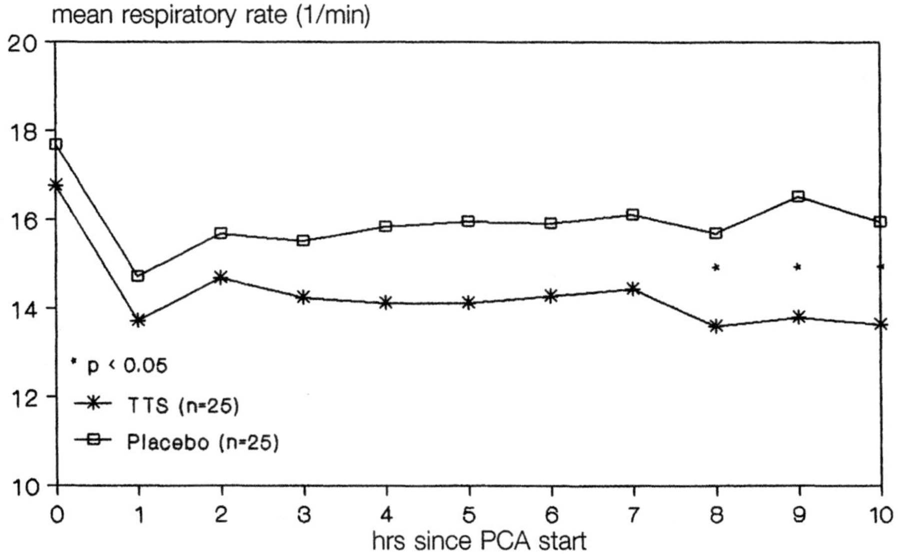

Fig. 4. Mean respiratory rates during PCA

h after initiation of PCA (Fig. 4). No respiratory depression requiring treatment developed in any patient.

Side effects were not statistically different for the two groups (Table 7). No observations on urinary retention could be made since all patients had urinary

Table 6. Retrospective pain scores

Pain score	TTS fentanyl	TTS placebo	Significance
VRS (0–5)	1.36 ± 0.95	1.60 ± 1.26	n.s.
VAS (0–100)	33.6 ± 23.4	37.2 ± 22.9	n.s.

Table 7. Number of patients experiencing side effects

Side effect	TTS fentanyl	TTS placebo
Sedation	20	20
Sweating	13	13
Nausea	14	10
Vomiting	4	2
Dizziness	3	3
Headache	1	2
Euphoria	0	2
Dysphoria	0	1
Local erythema	5	0
Local itching	1	1

catheters inserted. Sedation, as frequently reported, was generally described as pleasant. All patients were easily arousable. Taking into account that a prophylactic antiemetic had been given, postoperative nausea occurred mostly in a mild form and was easily controlled with droperidol.

Discussion

Transdermal drug administration is a relatively new concept designed to produce – after a gradual rise – constant plasma concentrations for a long period of time. It has already been tested for a variety of therapeutic agents including cardiovascular drugs, hormones, and antiemetics [1, 2, 4, 7, 8, 16, 28, 30]. The transdermal systems TTS fentanyl (Alza Corporation, Palo Alto, CA, USA) with delivery rates of 25, 50, 75, and 100 µg/h have been evaluated in numerous clinical investigations with patients suffering from acute [3, 5, 6, 9–11, 14, 23] and chronic pain [20, 25]. Transdermal fentanyl pharmacokinetics have been well documented by several investigators [3, 9–11, 14, 17, 20, 23, 24, 29]. The plasma concentrations reported ranged from 1 to 2 ng/ml 4–8 h after application of TTS fentanyl. The concentrations are in accordance with the minimum effective fentanyl concentrations (MEC) reported by Lehmann et al. after postoperative PCA studies [18, 19].

It was assumed that TTS fentanyl, with a delivery rate of 75 µg/h, applied 8 h prior to surgery should maintain postoperative plasma fentanyl concentrations at approximately the therapeutic threshold. Only a small amount of additional intravenous (PCA-) fentanyl should then be necessary to make the patients comfortable.

Patients from the placebo group self-administered fentanyl at the rate of 0.93 ± 0.46 µg/kg h. This quantity is more than the 0.46 µg/kg h reported by Lehmann et al. for abdominal and orthopedic patients recovering from neuroleptanalgesia [19], and the 0.79 µg/kg h for gynecological patients [18]. Fentanyl dosages of 0.75–0.86 µg/kg h were reported for abdominal surgery patients by Kay [15], Suttmann et al. [26], Rosenberg et al. [22] and Gourlay et al. [12], whereas even higher dosages of 1.03–1.38 µg/kg h were published by Moller et al. [21], Welchew [31] and Hackl et al. [13]. Although the reasons for these differences remain to be clarified, the administered opiate dosage for premedication and/or intraoperative analgesia seems to be important for the postoperative analgesic demand.

Patients with TTS fentanyl required significantly less operative and postoperative fentanyl than patients who had received TTS placebo (Fig. 2, Table 5), although both had virtually unlimited access to intravenous fentanyl supplementation. Considering the differences between the actual pain scores, retrospective pain scores did not show any difference between the groups.

It was supposed that the *total* amount of fentanyl taken would be about the same in both groups. Presumably the placebo group would require considerably more fentanyl intravenously than the verum group. In fact they required less fentanyl during PCA than had been predicted. Remarkably no patient demanded the maximum fentanyl dose, although patients in the TTS placebo group reported more pain during PCA than the patients in the TTS fentanyl group. Rowbotham et al. reported similar findings with patients recovering from abdominal surgery [23]. The reasons for this finding are not yet clear. Further investigation of this phenomenon with more detailed assessment of pain and tolerance to it is required, perhaps in cooperation with psychologists.

The present study demonstrates that the transdermal system TTS fentanyl can achieve a certain analgesic effect in patients recovering from major urological surgery. This may serve as a basis for postoperative pain relief. When, however, patients are also offered intravenous PCA, it becomes evident that TTS fentanyl alone (in the dose range studied) is not optimal, since all patients self-administered further doses of fentanyl (Fig. 1).

It seems unwise to recommend TTS with higher delivery rates for postoperative pain management for several reasons: Firstly, postoperative pain has been recognized as extremely variable; some patients seem to need only rather low analgesic doses or even no analgesics at all. Secondly, opiate-induced respiratory depression is thought to occur only with an overdose; prophylactic fentanyl delivered at rates higher than needed by individual patients is likely to induce dangerous respiratory complications. In order to prevent respiratory depression, intravenous titration of the analgesic is highly recommended in pain states with variable and time-dependent intensities. Thirdly, fentanyl is absorbed from the TTS to an intracutaneous depot from where systemic absorption takes place. Should signs of an overdose become apparent, removal of the TTS does not stop the fentanyl absorption immediately. The inverse connection between the state of vigilance and an opiate overdose is well established. Thus increasing sedation is likely to convert a previously well-tolerated dose into an overdose. When this occurs it is often necessary to stop postoperative analgesic delivery immediately. With a cutaneous fentanyl depot this is virtually impossible, leaving intravenous naloxone as the only alternative.

Although during the present study no serious adverse effects were observed (particularly no clinically relevant respiratory depression occurred), continuous patient monitoring is necessary when opiates are administered prophylactically.

In summary, TTS fentanyl (with a delivery rate of 75 μg/h) proved to provide beneficial analgesic effects in postoperative urological patients, although additional intravenous fentanyl was required by all patients. The transdermal system can only be recommended for basal postoperative pain relief and must be supplemented individually.

References

1. Aronson JK, Sear JW (1986) Transdermal hyoscine (scopolamine) and postoperative vomiting. Anaesthesia 41: 1–3
2. Bals-Pratsch M, Knuth UA, Yoon YD, Nieschlag E (1986) Transdermal testosterone substitutioned therapy for male hypogonadism. Lancet 1: 943–945
3. v. Bormann B, Ratthey K, Schwedtlick G, Schneider C, Müller H, Hempelmann G (1988) Postoperative Schmerztherapie durch transdermales Fentanyl. Anaesth Intensivther Notfallmed 23: 3–8
4. Buchkremer G, Bents H, Minneker E, Opitz K (1988) Langfristige Effekte einer Kombination von transdermaler Nikotinzufuhr mit Verhaltenstherapie zur Raucherentwöhnung. Nervenarzt 59: 488–490
5. Caplan RA, Ready LB, Oden RV, Matsen FA, Nessly ML, Olsson GL (1989) Transdermal fentanyl for postoperative pain management. JAMA 261: 1036–1039
6. Caplan RA, Southam M (1990) Transdermal drug delivery and its application to pain control. Adv Pain Res Ther 14: 233–240
7. Chetkowski RJ, Meldrum DR, Steingold KA, Randle D, Lu JK, Eggena P, Hershman JM, Alkjaersig NK, Fletcher AP, Judd HL (1986) Biologic effects of transdermal estradiol. N Engl J Med 314: 1615–1620
8. Chien YW, Piscataway NJ (1984) Pharmaceutical considerations of transdermal nitroglycerin delivery: The various approaches. Am Heart J 108: 207–216
9. Duthie DJR, Rowbotham DJ, Wyld R, Henderson PD, Nimmo WS (1988) Plasma fentanyl concentrations during transdermal delivery of fentanyl to surgical patients. Br J Anaesth 60: 614–618
10. Gourlay GK, Kowalski SR, Plummer JL, Cherry DA, Gaukroger P, Cousins MJ (1989) The transdermal administration of fentanyl in the treatment of postoperative pain: pharmacokinetics and pharmacodynamic effects. Pain 37: 193–202
11. Gourlay GK, Kowalski SR, Plummer JL, Cherry DA, Szekely SM, Mather LE, Owen H, Cousins MJ (1990) The efficacy of transdermal fentanyl in the treatment of postoperative pain: a double blind comparison of fentanyl and placebo systems. Pain 40: 21–28
12. Gourlay GK, Kowalski SR, Plummer JL, Cousins MJ, Armstrong PJ (1988) Fentanyl blood concentration-analgesic response relationship in the treatment of postoperative pain. Anesth Analg 67: 329–337
13. Hackl W, Fitzal S, Lackner F, Weindlmayr-Goettel M (1986) Vergleich von Fentanyl und Tramadol zur Schmerzbehandlung mittels On-demand-Analgesie-Computer in der frühen postoperativen Phase. Anaesthesist 35: 665–671
14. Holley FO, van Steennis CV (1988) Postoperative analgesia with fentanyl: pharmacokinetics and pharmacodynamics of constant rate i.v. and transdermal delivery. Br J Anaesth 60: 608–613
15. Kay B (1981) Postoperative pain relief. Use of an on-demand analgesia computer (ODAC) and a comparison of the rate of use of fentanyl and alfentanil. Anaesthesia 36: 949–951
16. Lasagna L, Greenblatt DJ (1986) More than skin deep: transdermal drug-delivery systems. N Engl J Med 314: 1638–1639
17. Latasch L, Lüders S (1989) Transdermal fentanyl against postoperative pain. Acta Anaesthesiol Belg 40: 113–119
18. Lehmann KA (1990) Patient-controlled analgesia for postoperative pain. Adv Pain Res Ther 14:297–324
19. Lehmann KA, Heinrich C, van Heiss R (1988) Balanced anaesthesia and patient-controlled postoperative analgesia with fentanyl: minimum effective concentrations, accumulation and acute tolerance. Acta Anaesthesiol Belg 39: 11–23
20. Miser AW, Narang PK, Dothage JA, Young RC, Sindelar W, Miser JS (1989) Transdermal fentanyl for pain control in patients with cancer. Pain 37:15–21

21. Moller IW, Dinesen K, Sondergard S, Knigge U, Kehlet H (1988) Effect of patient-controlled analgesia on plasma catecholamine, cortisol and glucose concentrations after cholecystectomy. Br J Anaesth 61: 160–164
22. Rosenberg PH, Heino A, Scheinin B (1984) Comparison of intramuscular analgesia, intercostal block, epidural morphine and on-demand i.v. fentanyl in the control of pain after upper abdominal surgery. Acta Anaesthesiol Scand 28: 603–607
23. Rowbotham DJ, Wyld R, Peacock JE, Duthie DJR, Nimmo WS (1989) Transdermal fentanyl for the relief of pain after upper abdominal surgery. Br J Anaesth 63: 56–59
24. Sebel PS, Barrett CW, Kirk CJC, Heykants J (1987) Transdermal absorption of fentanyl and sufentanil in man. Eur J Pharmacol 32: 529–531
25. Simmonds MA, Blain C, Richenbacher J, Southam MA (1988) A new approach to the administration of opiates: TTS (fentanyl) in the management of pain in patients with cancer. J Pain Sympt Manag 3: S18
26. Suttmann H, Juhl G, Dworzak H, Ebentheuer H (1988) Patientenkontrollierte Analgesie. Eine technische Spielerei oder eine Bereicherung der Schmerztherapie? Anaesthesist 37: 543–550
27. Tamsen A (1985) Prominject. In: Harmer M, Rosen M, Vickers MD (eds) Patient-controlled analgesia. Blackwell Scientific Publications, London, pp 92–93
28. Uppington J, Dunnet J, Blogg CE (1986) Transdermal hyoscine and vomiting. Anaesthesia 41: 16–20
29. Varvel JR, Shafer SL, Hwang SS, Coen PA, Stanski DR (1989) Absorption characteristics of transdermally administered fentanyl. Anesthesiology 70: 928–934
30. Weber MA, Drayer JIM, McMahon FG, Hamburger R, Shah AR, Kirk LN (1984) Transdermal administration of clonidine for treatment of high blood pressure. Arch Intern Med 144: 1211–1213
31. Welchew EA (1983) On-demand analgesia. A double blind comparison of on-demand intravenous fentanyl with regular intramuscular morphine. Anaesthesia 8: 19–25

Part V. Cancer Pain Management with TTS Fentanyl

Clinical Experience

D. ZECH, S. GROND, and J. LYNCH

Introduction

It is common knowledge among specialists that strong opioids play a major role in cancer pain management, and over the last years many reports supporting this opinion have been published [24–26, 28]. In one of our studies, strong opioids were used in more than half of 45000 treatment days with analgesics in 1070 cancer patients [28]. Another study demonstrated that more than two-thirds of 401 patients required these compounds in the final stage of malignant disease, i.e., in the last days and hours of life [10]. Although we know from an inpatient study that one-third of the patients need parenteral drug administration for different reasons at some time during treatment [27, 29], in only 6% of 55000 treatment days was sc or iv administration necessary in those 1070 patients already mentioned [28]. However, the situation is totally different in the 401 dying patients, almost half of whom received parenterally administered analgesics during the last days and hours of life [10].

Besides pain there are many other symptoms presenting in the terminal cancer patient that can impede effectiveness of oral drug administration and in turn lead to decreased bioavailability of analgesics. Anorexia, nausea, dysphagia, vomiting, and other gastrointestinal dysfunctions are very common symptoms in our patients not only on admission, but also during the course of treatment [8, 28]. Although the great majority of these symptoms are cancer-related, it is also true that oral administration of analgesics, and expecially opioids, can aggravate some of them. The usual alternative routes of administration today are continuous sc, iv, or spinal infusion by computerized pumps [2–5, 17, 18]. During the search for a simpler and less invasive mode of administration for these patients (in our experience suppositories are not very useful for long-term treatment in most of the patients), the transdermal application was found to offer an interesting and novel alternative.

The first trial with this new approach in cancer pain management was presented by Simmonds and coworkers at the 2nd International Congress on

This work was supported by a grant from Stada Arzneimittel AG.

Cancer Pain in New York in 1988 [22]. Their report concerned 16 patients who were first titrated with oral morphine to a stable dose and than converted to TTS.

A similar design was used by Richard Payne, who presented his results with TTS in 39 terminal cancer patients during a satellite symposium held at the VIth World Congress on Pain in Adelaide 1990 [19]. He described a 1-week prestudy stabilization phase with oral morphine to achieve satisfactory pain relief.

Angela Miser and coworkers, who recently published a report on five patients in the *Journal of Pain,* used their experience with the continuous intravenous infusion of fentanyl in the control of cancer pain to propose a different approach to dose finding [16]. Patients were initially given a continuous intravenous infusion of fentanyl at 0.5–1 μg/kg h. The dose was then adjusted to the lowest infusion rate yielding satisfactory analgesia as defined by a visual analogue scale (VAS) score below 35 mm. Once satisfactory pain relief had been achieved, TTS was applied to deliver the same microgram dosage rounded off to the closest 25 μg.

Materials and Methods

Overview

Bearing these reports in mind, as well as our positive previous experience with the use of patient-controlled analgesia (PCA) in the management of postoperative pain [12, 14, 15], we decided to perform a pilot study with 20 inpatients to investigate the use of PCA for dose titration and to combine rapid pain reduction with constant parenteral drug delivery by TTS.

Drug Administration and Procedure

Initially a 24 h period of i.v. fentanyl self-titration administered by a Deltec PCA pump (Pharmacia GmbH, Ratingen, Germany) was used for dose finding. Based on the titrated dose and a conversion table, the required daily dose of transdermal fentanyl was calculated and the first TTS administered on the 2nd day. This patch remained in place for 72 h, while iv fentanyl was available for a further 48 h. The size of a second TTS applied from day 5 to 7 was adjusted according to the amount of supplementary iv doses required on the second day of transdermal administration. From day 4 to 7 sc morphine was available for breakthrough pain on a p.r.n. basis. Fifteen patients were reconverted to oral or parenteral morphine on day 8 as indicated by the study protocol, whereas five continued with TTS for up to 34 days. Standardized adjuvant drugs, i.e., nonopioid analgesics, antiemetics and laxatives were provided, and patients with simultaneous chemotherapy or surgery were excluded. Only patients in the first 2 weeks of radiotherapy were included.

Collected data

Pain, mood, general state of health, activity, disease symptoms and adverse effects were assessed daily by patient-completed VASs. Vital functions were monitored four times daily. Pain relief was assessed on the first and fourth days using a 5-point scale covering 0%–100% pain relief. Plasma fentanyl concentrations were checked daily using a radioimmunoassay technique.

Results

Demographic Data and Prestudy Conditions

Ten women and ten men (mean age: 57 years) with different tumour sites were included in this study; three of these patients had cancers of the oral cavity or nasopharynx and four had gastrointestinal malignancies (Table 1).

Fourteen of them suffered from soft tissue, bone or visceral pain, i.e., nociceptor pain, eight from neuropathic pain and two from combinations of these. All patients had already been treated following the WHO analgesic guidelines prior to the study. Sixteen patients received oral morphine in doses

Table 1. Demographic data

Patient no.	Age (years)	Weight (kg)	Height (cm)	Sex (M/F)	Cancer diagnosis	Prior treatment (WHO step)
1	60	58	162	F	Non-Hodgkin's lymphoma	2
2	63	77	181	M	Stomach	2
3	67	60	168	F	Colon	3
4	50	60	168	M	Nasopharynx	3
5	40	58	190	M	Floor of mouth	3
6	48	64	165	F	Breast	3
7	41	59	155	F	Breast	2
8	46	78	184	M	Colon	3
9	65	53	161	F	Bladder	3
10	66	97	185	M	Kidney	3
11	53	65	180	M	Floor of mouth	3
12	65	90	174	M	Bladder	3
13	59	70	158	F	Breast	3
14	68	97	181	M	Prostate	3
15	44	90	153	F	Breast	3
16	66	84	182	M	Non-Hodgkin's lymphoma	3
17	64	82	155	F	Breast	3
18	62	51	153	F	Parotid gland	3
19	64	84	182	M	Kidney	3
20	44	79	170	F	Rectum	3

ranging from 30 to 200 mg/day (mean dose 98 mg/day) for an average period of 20 days. One patient received a sc morphine infusion of 165 mg/day for 9 days and three patients were unsatisfactorily controlled with tramadol, a weak opioid which we use as a substitute for codeine in WHO step 2.

Fentanyl Requirement and Plasma Fentanyl Concentrations

The mean daily PCA fentanyl dose amounted to 1.5 mg during the first 24 h and decreased on days 2 and 3 (with the onset of TTS action) to 0.8 and 0.7 mg respectively (Fig. 1).

The mean daily TTS dose during days 2 to 4 was again 1.5 mg, whereas the additional iv fentanyl requirements on day 3 were the basis for an increased mean TTS dose of almost 2 mg during days 5 to 7 (Fig. 2).

The mean plasma fentanyl concentrations obtained in 15 patients amounted to 1 ng/ml during the first 24 h PCA phase and increased to 1.4 and 1.2 ng respectively on days 2 and 3, before decreasing to values below 1 ng/ml on day 4. The plasma fentanyl concentration curve from days 5 to 7 shows a comparable shape but on a lower level. A decline of the fentanyl concentration curve for both patches on the 3rd day of transdermal administration was noticed. There was still a plasma fentanyl concentration of 0.4 on day 8 when most of the patients had already been reconverted to morphine (Fig. 3).

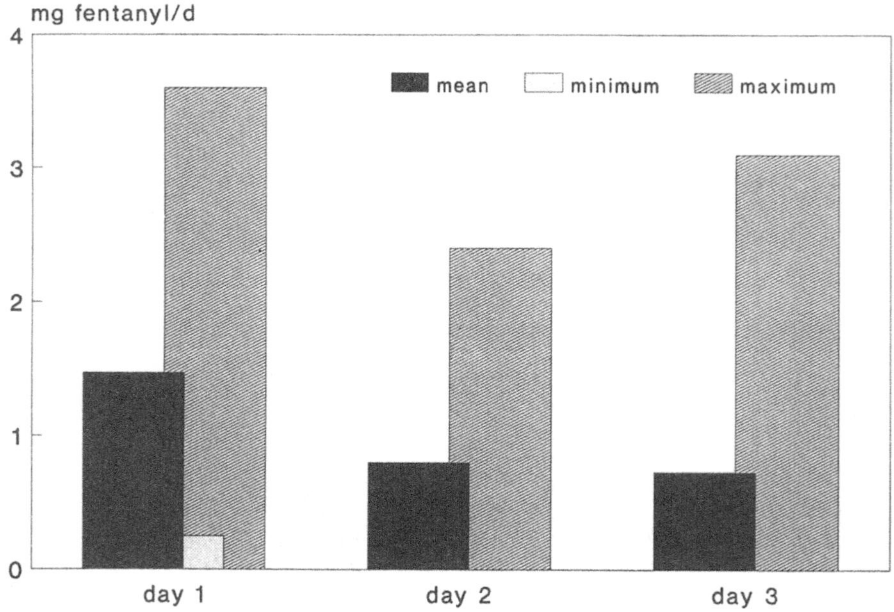

Fig. 1. Mean daily PCA fentanyl doses during days 1–3 (n = 20)

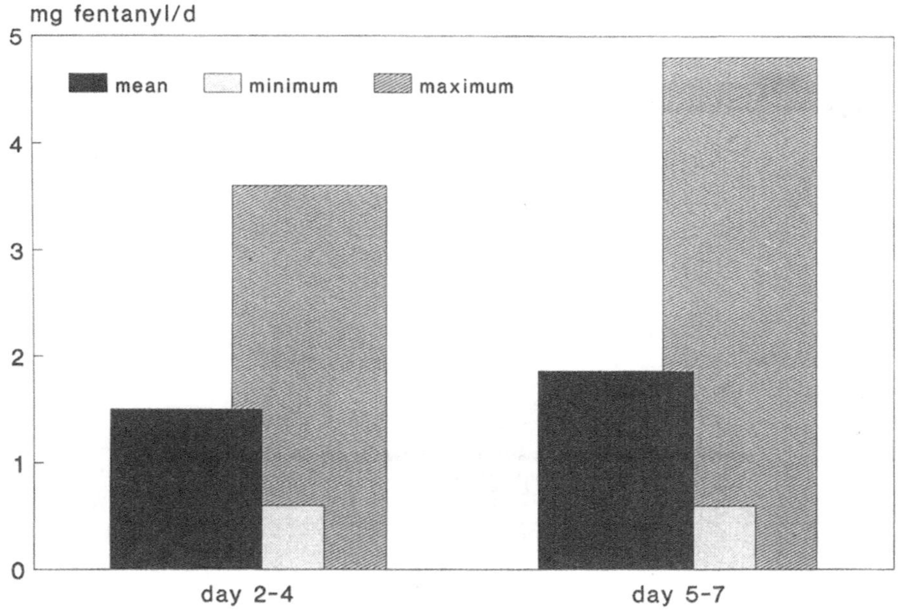

Fig. 2. Mean daily TTS Fentanyl doses during days 2–7 (n = 20)

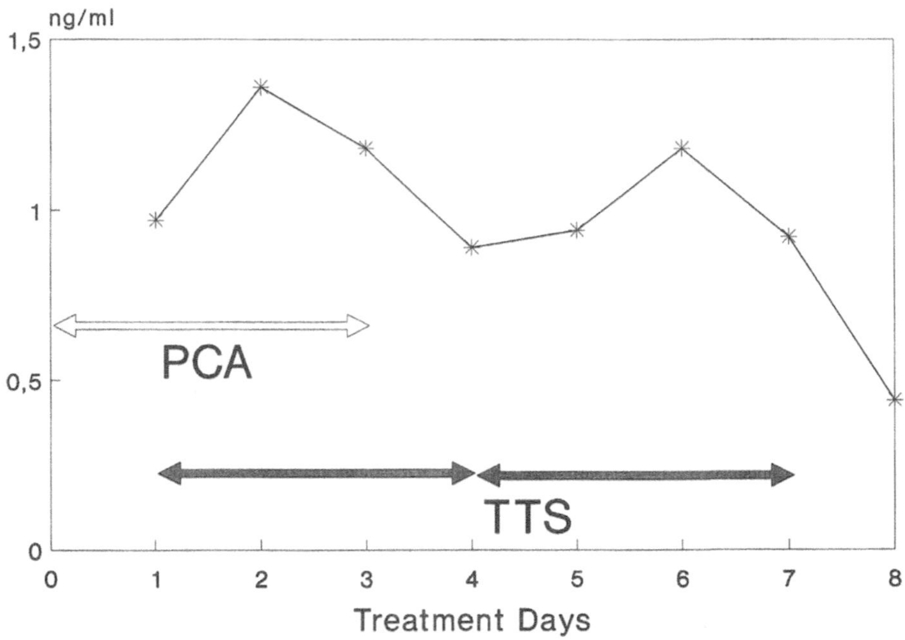

Fig. 3. Mean plasma fentanyl concentrations during days 1–8 (n = 15)

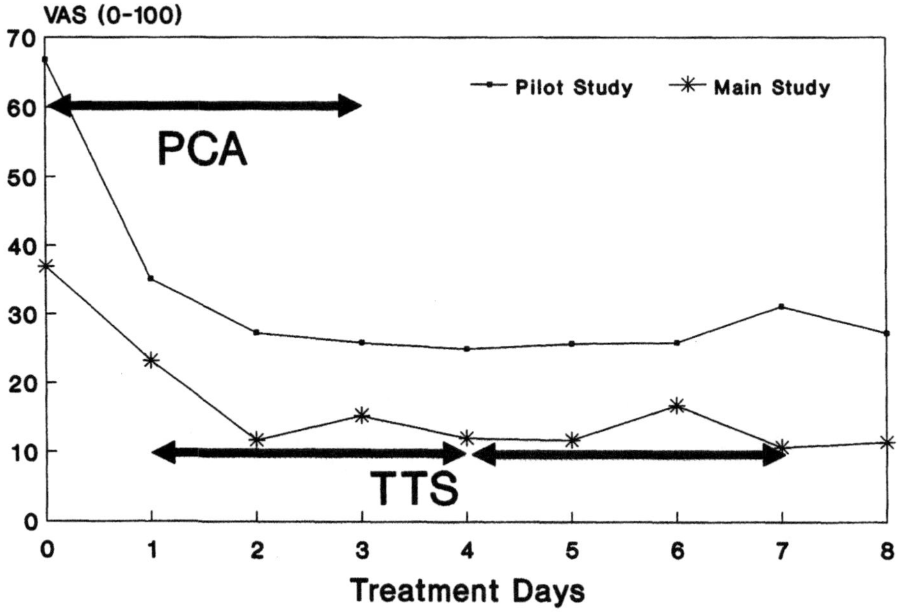

Fig. 4. Mean daily VAS scores: comparison of pilot study ($n = 20$) and preliminary results of the main study ($n = 15$); in the main study, conversion ratio from iv to transdermal route was increased by 1/3

Pain Report and Supplementary Morphine doses

The mean daily VAS scores decreased from 68 mm to 35 mm on day 1 and further to values around 25 mm from days 2 to 6 before they increased again to 31 on day 7 (Fig. 4).

The mean supplementary morphine doses amounted to 25 mg/day on day 4 and decreased on days 5 and 6 to 14 mg/day, before increasing again to 20 mg/day (Fig. 5).

A combination of relatively low plasma fentanyl concentrations and relatively high supplementary morphine doses was noted on days 4 and 7. By way of contrast the mean pain relief scores increased from 10% on day 1 to 44% on day 4.

Side Effects

Severe side effects such as clinically apparent respiratory depression or significant changes in blood pressure or heart rate could not be observed throughout the study. Four patients presented with a slight and very transient erythema after removing the patch, and one patient developed minor pustules, which resolved spontaneously after a few days.

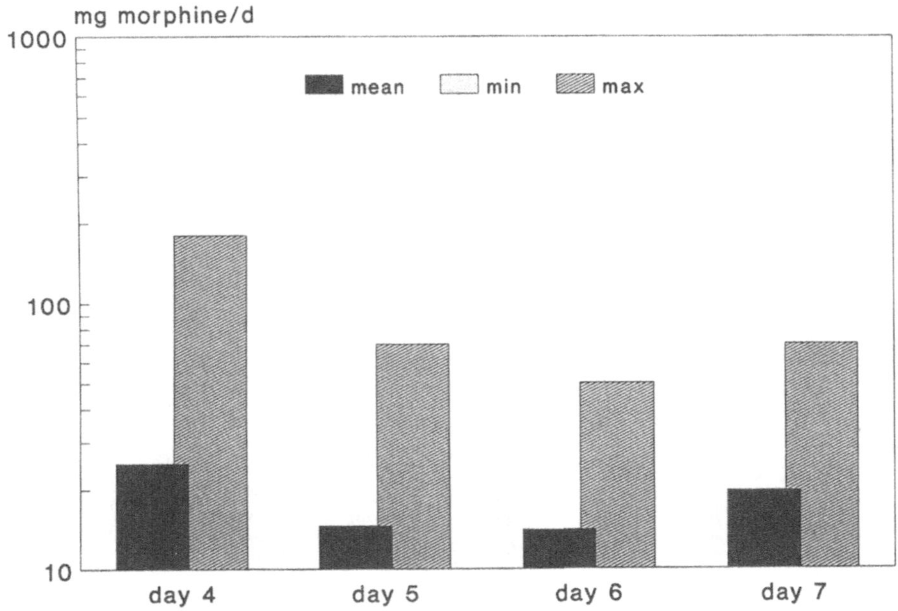

Fig. 5. Mean daily sc morphine doses during days 4–7 (n = 20)

In comparison with the prestudy situation there was a slight increase in the number of patients who presented with constipation, nausea and vomiting (Fig. 6).

However, in the majority of the patients these symptoms were believed to be cancer-related. If we look more closely at one of those symptoms, for instance nausea, we find a moderate level of VAS scores for nausea decreasing in the first part of the study and increasing again in the second part, but to a lower level than initially. This observation, as well as the fluctuating numbers of patients presenting with this symptom throughout the study, may not be considered typical of opioid side effects (Fig. 7).

Other major symptoms were dry mouth, sweating, drowsiness and dizziness (Fig. 8). If we focus again on two of these symptoms, drowsiness and dizziness, we find that the number of patients with the former changed from day to day and the degree of drowsiness decreased rapidly during the study period (Fig. 9). The symptom of dizziness showed quite a different picture. Fewer patients presented with dizziness after entering the study, but the dizziness increased to a higher, though still moderate and clinically acceptable, level (Fig. 10).

To summarize, major side effects were constipation and dryness of the mouth, which may have also been influenced by the concomitant application of nonsteroidals and antiemetics.

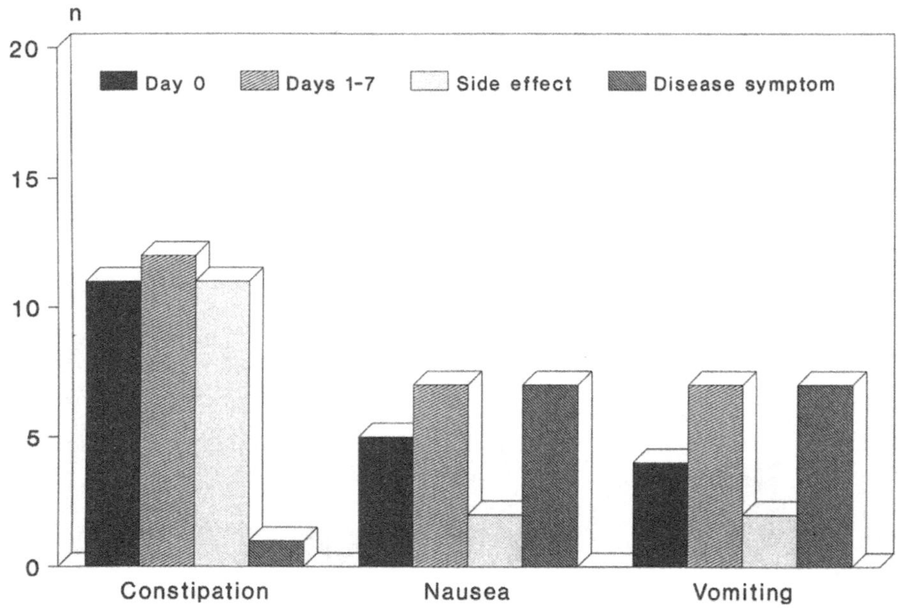

Fig. 6. Major side effects and disease symptoms: a slight increase in the frequency of gastrointestinal symptoms during TTS could be observed; these were thought to be mainly cancer-related

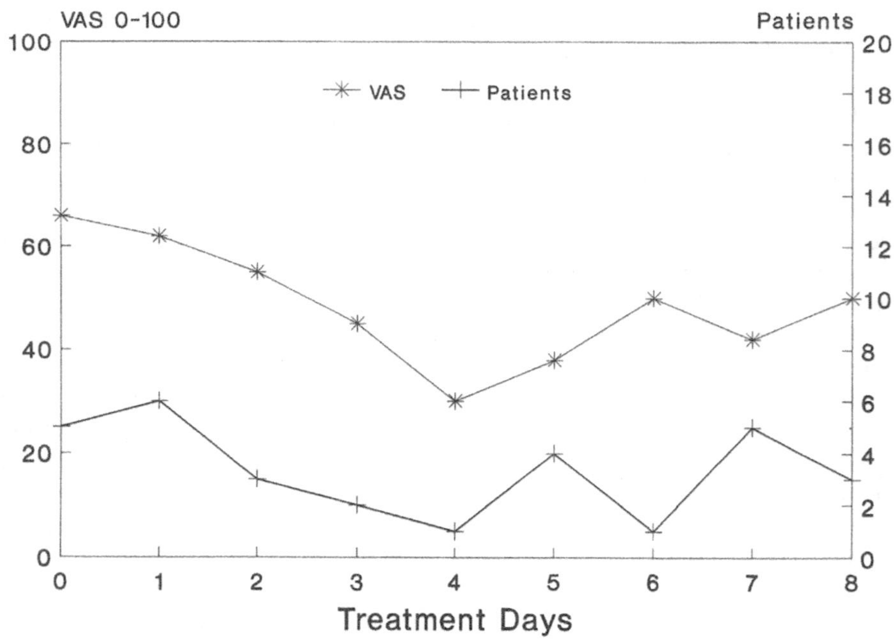

Fig. 7. Patients with the symptom of nausea. The number of patients from days 0–8 and their mean visual analogue scores are plotted here. The fluctuating curves may not be considered typical for purely adverse effects

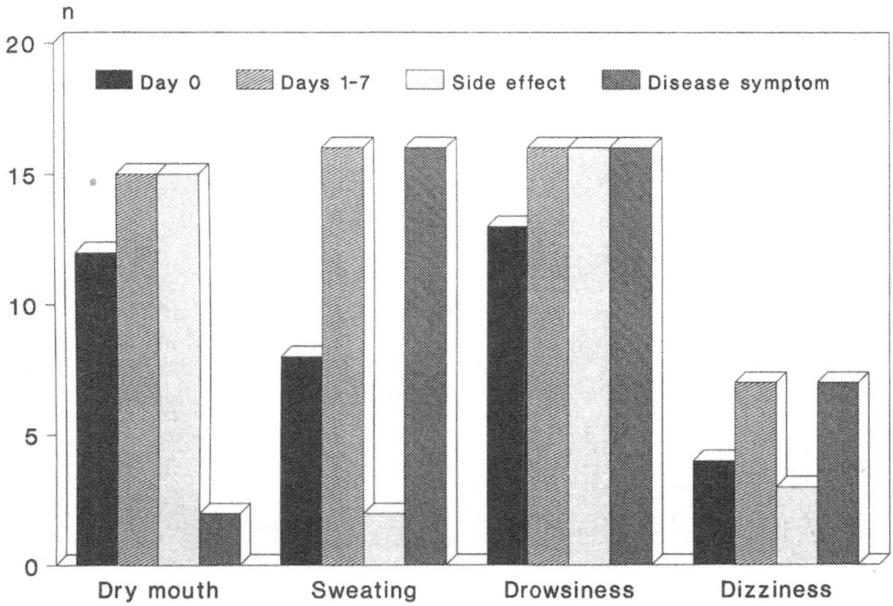

Fig. 8. Major side effects and disease symptoms: a considerable increase in sweating could be observed. Generally the differentiation between side effects and disease symptoms was difficult and sometimes impossible. In these cases the symptom was judged to be influenced by both disease and drug treatment

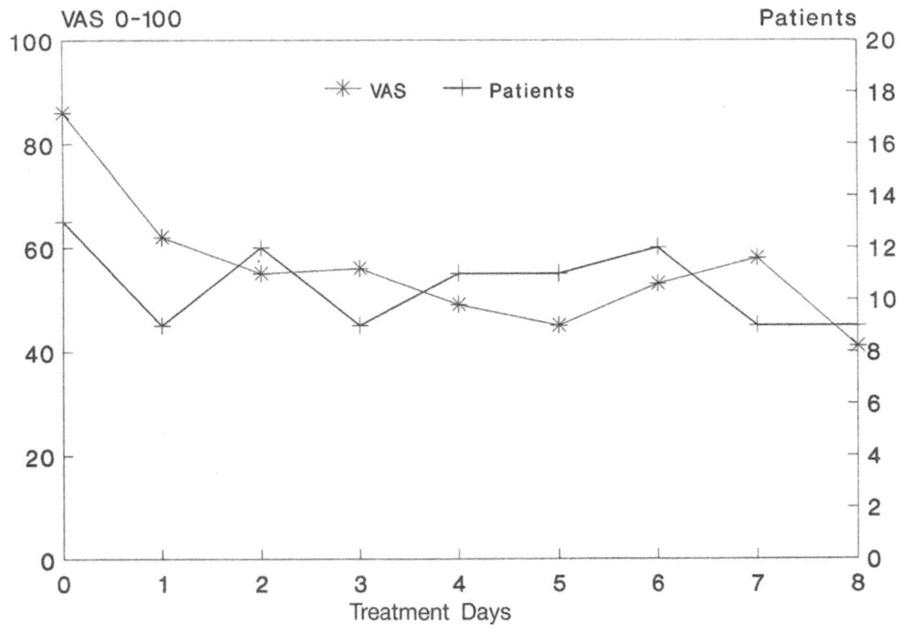

Fig. 9. Patients with the symptom of drowsiness. The number of patients from days 0–8, and their mean visual analogue scores, are plotted here. A substantial decrease in the VAS scores (degree of drowsiness) could be observed, whereas the number of patients was almost unchanged

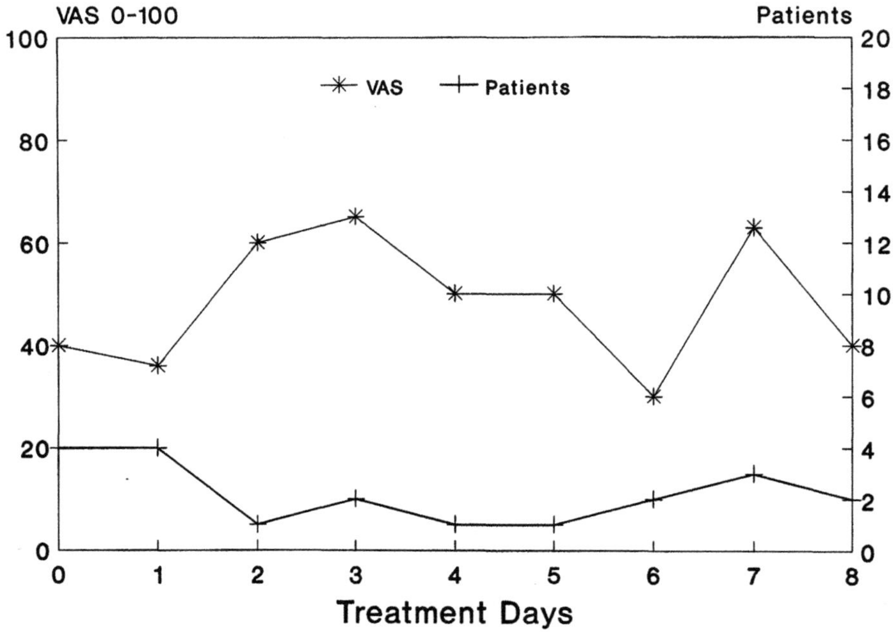

Fig. 10. Patients with the symptom of dizziness. The number of patients from days 0–8, and their mean visual analogue scores, are plotted here. An increased degree of dizziness (VAS scores) is connected with a decreased number of patients presenting with dizziness

Mood, General State of Health and Activity Level

There was a modest increase in the VAS scores of mood and general state of health, whereas the activity level did not change very much (Fig. 11).

Prolonged Treatment in Five Patients

Because of the excellent patient compliance and acceptance of the transdermal route, we decided to continue TTS as long as the patients remained in hospital. After obtaining the consent of our national drug administration, five patients were continued for periods of 20–34 days. Most of these patients had quite stable fentanyl requirements during the transdermal administration (Fig. 12). The highest fentanyl dose of more than 7 mg daily was recorded in the particularly extreme case of one patient with a highly malignant and widespread tumor of the parotid gland, who presented with diffuse skeletal metastases and accompanying pathological fractures of ribs and vertebral bodies and infiltration of the jugular foramen on both sides. The VAS scores of all five patients ranged between 0 and 40 mm, representing excellent to moderate pain control with the exception of the aforementioned patient (Fig. 13).

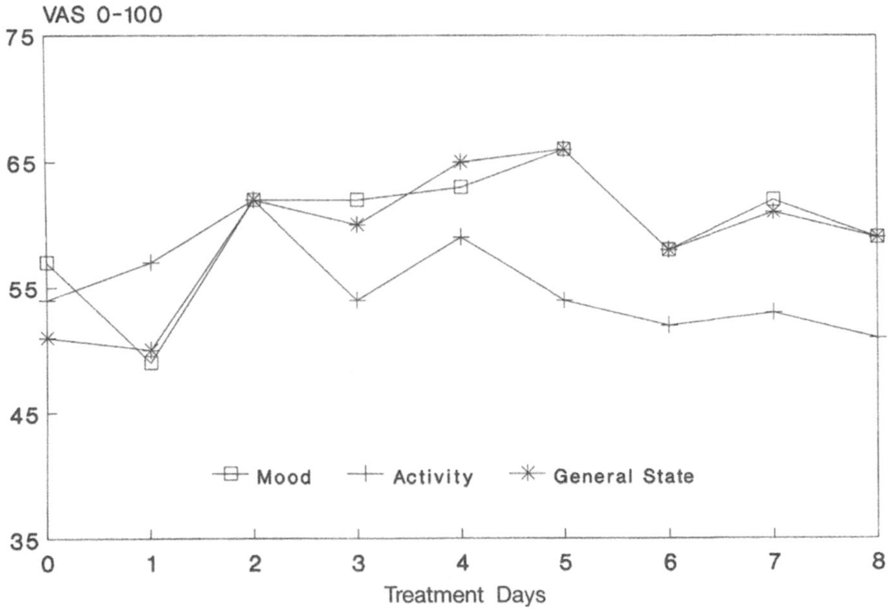

Fig. 11. Patient-completed mean visual analogue scores for mood, activity and general state of health from days 0–8. A modest increase for mood and general state of health and an unchanged activity level resulted

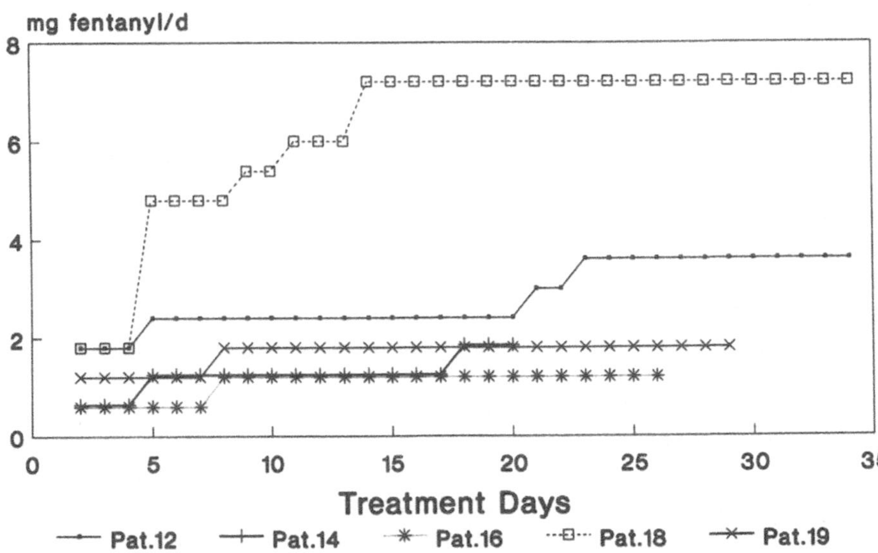

Fig. 12. Daily TTS Fentanyl doses for five patients with prolonged TTS treatment. Four patients presented with quite stable fentanyl requirements, whereas the fifth patient (pat. 18) required more than 7 mg/day due to a highly malignant and widespread carcinoma of the parotid gland

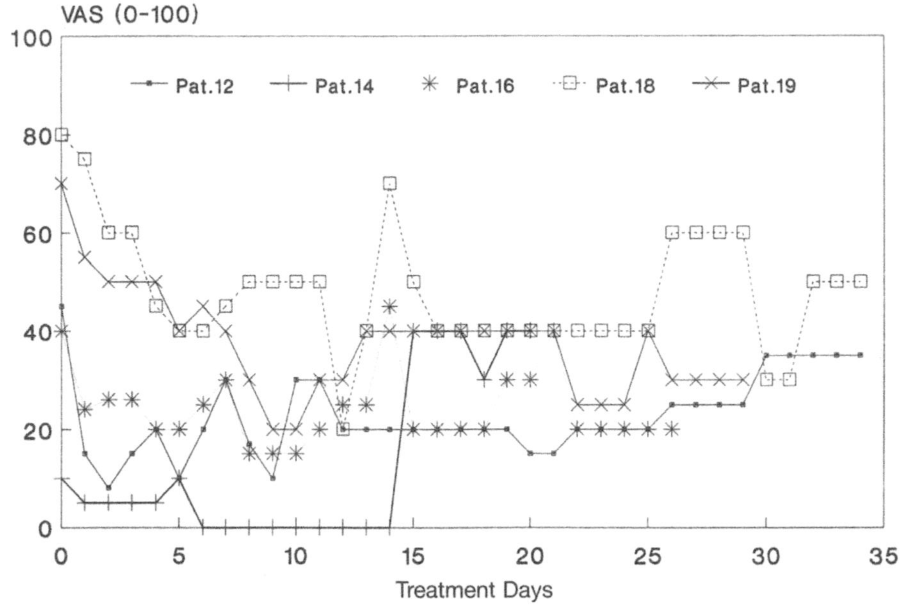

Fig. 13. Daily visual analogue pain scores for five patients with prolonged TTS treatment. In spite of a high fentanyl dose, the prescription of coanalgesics and high doses of additional morphine pain relief in patient 18 was unsatisfactory

The mean daily supplementary morphine dose was around 25 mg with high maximum doses once again being due to this extreme case.

Discussion

The first trial with TTS fentanyl in cancer pain management was performed by Simmonds and coworkers [22]. Sixteen patients were titrated with oral morphine to a stable dose and then converted to TTS. Immediate release morphine was available for breakthrough pain. The mean VAS score for pain at the time of morphine stabilization was 4.6 cm, and 1 month after the patients had started to wear the patch it was 3.2 cm. The median morphine stabilization dose was 180 mg/day and the median supplementary dose was 90 mg/day.

A similar design in 39 terminal cancer patients was used by Richard Payne [19]. He described a 1 week prestudy stabilization phase with oral morphine to achieve satisfactory pain relief. One month after initiating the study VAS pain intensity ratings decreased from 4.6 cm after the stabilization phase to 4.1 cm. The mean morphine stabilization dose was 120 mg daily and the median rescue dose was 105 mg/day. In the meantime, the groups of Payne and Simmonds have been pooled and their results presented together [20], i.e., the aforementioned eighteen patients are included in the total number of 39 patients.

Angela Miser and coworkers reported on five patients with TTS treatment using a different approach to dose finding [16]. Patients were begun on a continuous intravenous infusion of fentanyl at 0.5–1 µg/kg h. The dose was then adjusted to the lowest infusion rate yielding satisfactory analgesia as defined by a VAS score below 35 mm. Once satisfactory pain relief had been achieved, TTS was applied to deliver the same microgram dosage rounded off to the closest 25 µg. VAS scores prior to entrance into the study were not available, but all patients achieved good to excellent pain control, defined as VAS scores between 0 and 35 mm. The duration of the titration phase was only mentioned for one patient, where it lasted 48 h. Additional narcotic medications were not used, but one patient became somnolent and two patients developed respiratory depression which resolved when the fentanyl dose was reduced.

Proper dose finding is a vital step towards achieving an equilibrium between maximum pain relief and the occurrence of major side effects. Another important point is a quick and safe dose titration in terminal cancer patients, who should not lose much of their limited time for medical procedures in hospital or suffer from severe side effects.

The results reported by Payne and Simmonds demonstrate that quick and effective dose finding with oral and parenteral morphine is difficult to achieve, since pain relief was still unsatisfactory some 4 weeks into the study and supplementary morphine doses were high in comparison to the initial stabilization dose. Because of considerable interindividual variations in the bioavailability of oral morphine [21] and the variable equipotency that is reported for fentanyl in comparison with morphine [7, 11, 13, 23], this is not a surprising finding.

In the report by Miser et al. the duration of the titration phase was only mentioned for one patient. No information was given on pain scores prior to entrance into the study. Since three of the five patients showed signs of cerebral impairment (somnolence, respiratory depression) an overdose may be presumed. This might have been the consequence of a low basic pain intensity and an overtitration with fentanyl doses, which were initially based on body weight. The latter has not proved to be of much value in pain management [1, 6]. In our study dose titration using PCA resulted in quick and effective pain control within 48 h. Additionally, pain intensity scores were stable almost throughout the study period. Supplementary morphine doses were needed,, however, to a lesser extent when compared to the study of Payne and Simmonds. Severe side effects such as respiratory depression and somnolence did not occur.

The results in those five patients where TTS was continued after the test phase were not fully satisfactory because of unstable pain relief with episodes of "breakthrough pain" which resulted in increasing supplementary morphine doses. This might be partly due to a conversion ratio from iv to transdermal fentanyl that was too low.

Conclusions

In conclusion, this pilot study demonstrated the safety and usefulness of initial PCA in combination with TTS for cancer pain. The results indicate quick and effective pain relief; adverse effects played a minor role and could be controlled using adjuvant medication. Increasing VAS scores and supplementary morphine doses as well as decreasing plasma fentanyl concentrations on day 7 indicated that conversion ratios from iv to transdermal administration should be changed.

Preliminary Results of a New Inpatient and Outpatient Study

Since patients with head and neck cancers usually present with symptoms such as anorexia and dysphagia, which may also occur in the course of our therapy [9], we recently started a new in- and outpatient study (main study) on a total of 50 patients with head and neck cancers and gastrointestinal malignancies. The latter are also known to present with a higher rate of gastrointestinal symptoms. Following our experience with the pilot study, we increased the conversion ratio by one-third. In contrast to the pilot study, a time limit for the duration of therapy was not set. Preliminary results from 15 patients show that mean daily PCA fentanyl doses from days 1 to 3 were almost similar in these investigations with the exception of higher mean and maximum doses on days 2 and 3 in the main study. As a result of the increased conversion ratio the mean daily TTS fentanyl doses were significantly higher in these fifteen patients (Fig. 14).

The mean daily VAS scores decreased from 37 mm initially to values between 10 and 17 mm throughout the study and were significantly lower than those in the pilot study (Fig. 4). These superior results are supported by mean daily supplementary morphine doses ranging from 7 to 8 mg which decreased further on day 8 in comparison to a range of 14 to 25 mg/day in the pilot study (Fig. 15).

Our interpretation of the preliminary results would suggest that the increase of the conversion ratio contributed to this improvement. However, one common problem arose in individual patients with high fentanyl requirements as a result of this increased ratio. It may be extremely difficult to find suitable sites for patch application in individual patients (e.g., cachectic and bony patients, and patients with skin ulcerations) when skin sites have to be rotated with each application.

Acknowledgements. We wish to thank H. G. Dauer, B. Stollenwerk, T. Hinck, and H. Jung for their assistance in performing these studies.

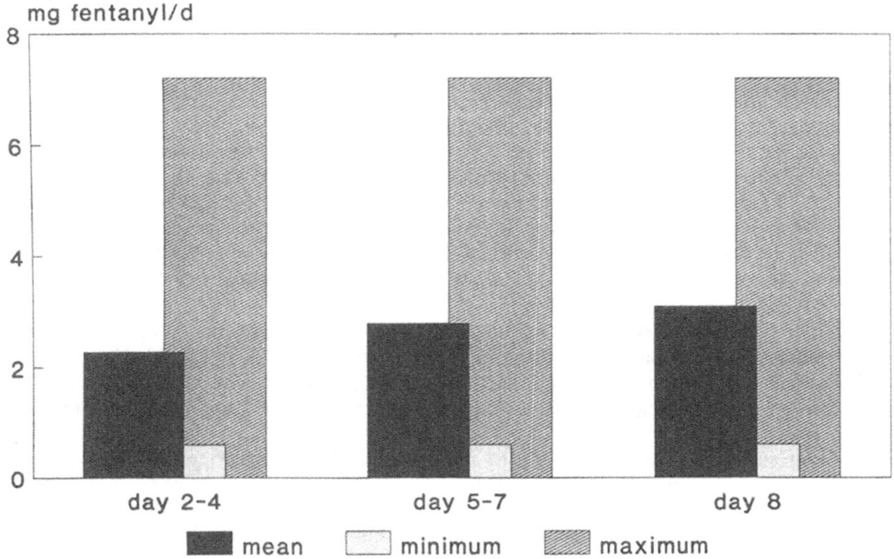

Fig. 14. Mean daily TTS fentanyl doses in 15 patients after increasing the conversion ratio by 1/3 (main study)

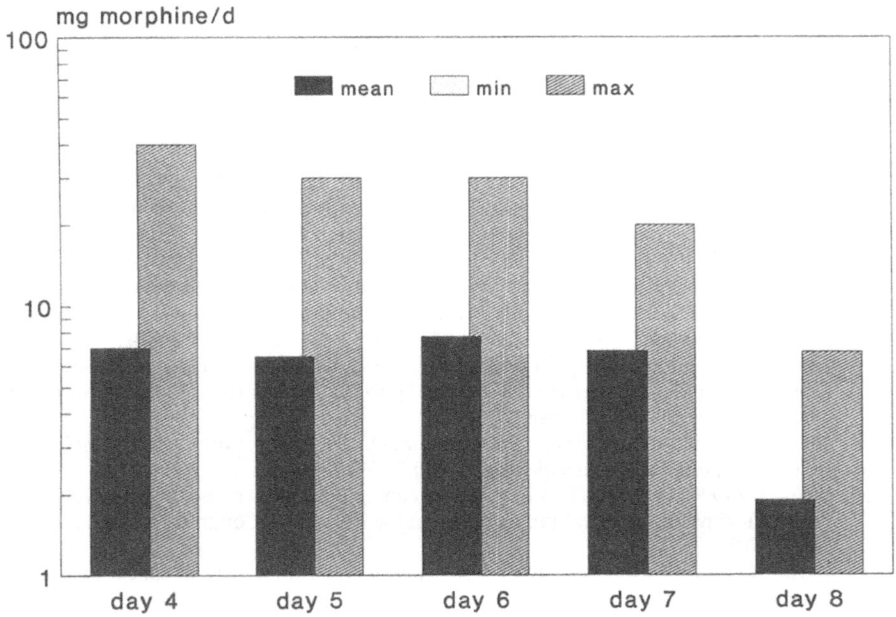

Fig. 15. Mean daily sc morphine doses in the main study with increased fentanyl conversion ratio

References

1. Burns JW, Hodsman NBA, McLintock TTC, Gillies GWA, Kenny GNC, McArdle CS (1989) The influence of patient characteristics on the requirements for postoperative analgesia. A reassessment using patient-controlled analgesia. Anaesthesia 44: 2–6
2. Campbell CF, Mason JB, Weiler JM (1983) Continuous subcutaneous infusion of morphine for the pain of terminal malignancy. Ann Intern Med 98, no. 1: 51–52
3. Citron ML, Johnston-Early A, Boyer M, Krsnow SH, Hood M, Cohen MH (1986) Patient-controlled analgesia for severe cancer pain. Arch Intern Med 146: 734–736
4. Coombs DW, Saunders RL, Fratkin JD, Jensen LE, Murphy CA (1986) Continuous intrathecal hydromorphone and clonidine for intractable cancer pain. J Neurosurg 64: 890–894
5. Coyle N, Mauskop A, Maggard J, Foley K (1986) Continuous subcutaneous infusions of opiates in cancer patients with pain. Oncol Nurs Forum 13, no. 4: 53–57
6. Ginsberg B, Cohen NA, Ossey KD, Glass PSA (1989) The use of PCA to assess the influence of demographic factors on analgesic requirements. Anesthesiology 71: A688
7. Gourlay GK, Kowalski SR, Plummer JL, Cousins MJ, Armstrong PJ (1988) Fentanyl blood concentration-analgesic response relationship in the treatment of postoperative pain. Anesth Analg 67: 329–337
8. Grond S, Zech D, Dahlmann H, Stobbe B, Lehmann KA (1990): Intractable cancer pain as a reason for referral. Analysis of pain etiology and previous drug treatment. Der Schmerz 4: 193–200
9. Grond S, Zech D, Meuser T, Stobbe B, Lehmann KA (1989) Schmerztherapie bei malignen Kopf-Hals-Tumoren – Erfahrungen mit dem Stufenplan der WHO. Anaesthesist 38 (Suppl) 1: 561
10. Grond S, Zech D, Meuser T, Stobbe B, Lehmann KA (1990) Cancer pain relief in dying patients. Pain (Suppl 5): S355
11. Hackl W, Fitzal S, Lackner F, Weindlmayr-Goettel M (1986) Vergleich von Fentanyl und Tramadol zur Schmerzbehandlung mittels On-Demand-Analgesie-Computer in der frühen postoperativen Phase. Anaesthesist 35: 665–671
12. Lehmann KA (1990) Patient-controlled analgesia for postoperative pain. Adv Pain Res Ther 14: 297
13. Lehmann KA (1991) Patient-controlled analgesia for postoperative pain. In: Benedetti C, Chapman R, Giron G (eds) Opioid analgesia: Recent advances in systemic administration. Advances in pain research and therapy: in press
14. Lehmann KA, Gerhard A, Horrichs-Haermeyer G, Zech D (1991) Postoperative patient-controlled analgesia with sufentanil. Analgesic efficacy and minimum effective concentrations. Acta Anaesthesiol Scand, 35: 221–226
15. Lehmann KA, Kratzenberg U, Schroeder-Bark B, Horrichs-Haermeyer G (1990) Postoperative patient-controlled analgesia with tramadol. Analgesic efficacy and minimum effective concentrations. Clin J Pain 6: 212–220
16. Miser AW, Narang PK, Dothage JA, Young RC, Sindelar W, Miser JS (1989) Transdermal fentanyl for pain control in patients with cancer. Pain 37: 15–21
17. Motsch J, Schüder G, Bier B (1987) Use of portable pumps for continuous intrathecal narcotics infusion. Anaesthesist 36: 391
18. Müller H, Lüben V, Zierski J, Hempelmann G (1988) Long term spinal opiate treatment. Acta Anaesthesiol Belg, Suppl 2, 39, 2: 83–86
19. Payne R (1990) Fentanyl TTS in terminal cancer pain. Abstracts of Symposium "New Opioid Techniques in Pain Management" at the VIth World Congress on Pain, Adelaide 1990, p 16
20. Payne R (1990) Experience with transdermal fentanyl in advanced cancer pain. Eur J Pain 11: 98–101
21. Säwe J, Dahlström B, Paalzow L, Rane A (1981) Morphine kinetics in cancer patients. Clin Pharmacol Ther 30: 629–635

22. Simmonds MA, Blain C, Richenbacher J, Southam MA (1988) A new approach to the administration of opiates: TTS (Fentanyl) in the management of pain in patients with cancer. J Pain Sympt Manag 3, 3: S18
23. Stoelting RK (1987) Pharmacology and physiology in anaesthetic practice. Lippincott, Philadelphia
24. Takeda F (1986) Results of field-testing in Japan of the WHO Draft Interim Guideline on Relief of Cancer Pain. The Pain Clinic 1, 2: 83–89
25. Ventafridda V, Tamburini M, Caraceni A, DeConno F, Naldi F (1987) A validation study of the WHO method for cancer pain relief. Cancer 59: 850–856
26. Walker VA, Hoskin PJ, Hanks GW, White ID (1988) Evaluation of WHO analgesic guidelines for cancer pain in a hospital-based palliative care unit. J Pain Sympt Manag 3, 3: 145–149
27. Zech D (1988) Schmerztherapie auf einer Palliativstation – ein Modellversuch. In: Peter K, Groh J (Hrsg) ZAK München 1987 Band III – Hauptthemen; Reihe Anaesthesiologie und Intensiv-Medizin Band 205, Springer Verlag, Berlin Heidelberg New York, pp 216–228
28. Zech D, Grond S, Schug SA, Meuser T, Stobbe B, Lehmann KA (1990) Pain control according to WHO guidelines in 1070 cancer patients. Résumés des Communications, 1er Congrès de l'association européenne de soins palliatifs, Paris, 17.–19. 10. 1990, p 137
29. Zech D, Schug SA (1988) Pain control in a palliative care unit (Poster). European Congress on Palliative Care, 23.–25. 4. 1988, Milan, Italy

Part VI. Other Transdermal Therapeutic Systems for Anesthesia and Pain Management

Local Anesthetics: Eutectic Mixture of Local Anesthetics

M. Y. Dubois

Introduction

All commonly available local anesthetics have poor skin penetration when applied topically. One of the main reasons is that a local anesthetic agent needs to be in its cationic form in order to block nerve conduction. But it is the uncharged base which penetrates and diffuses into the tissues after topical administration. It has been shown that an effective tissue penetration can be achieved by using an oil-in-water emulsion that combines a high concentration of local anesthetic base with a high water content [5]. If lidocaine is emulsified, it produces only 20% active substance in each emulsion droplet. If, on the other hand, lidocaine and prilocaine crystals are mixed, they will form a "eutectic" mixture that produces an emulsion droplet with about 80% of active local anesthetic substance. This is the basis of the composition of the EMLA (Eutectic Mixture of Local Anesthetics) cream, comprised of an equal amount of lidocaine and prilocaine with an emulsifier and a thickener; sodium hydroxide and water complete the formula (Table 1).

Testing in Volunteers

Evaluation of pain-relief using a model with laser-induced pain was made in a comparative study of EMLA with local injection of lidocaine by Arendt-

Table 1. Composition of EMLA cream (5%)

Ingredient	Quantity (g)
Lidocaine (base)	2.5 (107 mmol/l)
Prilocaine (base)	2.5 (113 mmol/l)
Arlatone 289*	1.9
Carbopol 934**	1.0
Sodium hydroxide 2M	7.2
Purified water	100.0

* Emulsifier
** Thickener

Nielsen and Bjerring [1]. These investigators were able to quantify three different parameters: the sensory threshold, the pain threshold, and the pain-evoked brain cortical response. Using this technique it was possible to distinguish between a pain block (where no pain was felt but other sensations were still perceived), and total sensory block, where the laser stimulus elicited no sensations of any kind. Lidocaine local injection produced total sensory block almost immediately. When the EMLA cream was applied for 15 min, both sensory and pain thresholds increased. Total sensory block was reached 20 min after removal of application for 80 min or immediately after removal of the cream after it was applied for 100 or 120 min. Pain block, on the other hand, was achieved 30 min after removal of the cream applied for 30 min as well as 15 min after removal of cream applied for 60 min and immediately after applications for 80, 100, or 120 min. Cortical responses evoked by thermal argon laser pulses applied to the dorsal area of the hand showed decreases in amplitude and increases in latency which reflected the decrease in perception of these stimuli. The same investigators [3] determined the depth and duration of skin analgesia to needle insertion after topical application of EMLA. They found that the depth of sensory and pain thresholds was related to the length of the application times. The maximum depth of analgesia was found to be approximately 5 mm and was observed 30 min after a 90 min application and during the 60 min period after a 120 min application for both sensory and pain thresholds. For applications shorter than 2 h, the depth of analgesia increased during the period after removal of the cream. Following a 30 min application of EMLA it was observed that a significant increase in pain threshold depth occurred 30 min before the sensory threshold depth increased, which suggests that lidocaine blocks transmission potential in small fibers before large fibers are themselves blocked [3]. In a further study [2], the same investigators studied the local vascular responses after skin application of EMLA by skin refractance spectroscopy and laser doppler blood flowmetry. They found a biphasic vascular response with an initial vascular constriction maximal 1½ h after the beginning of the application and a secondary vasodilation after 3 h. EMLA was tested together with other creams which all produced initial blanching, but only EMLA produced late erythema after 4 h of application. Finally, the effects of EMLA on tourniquet pain were studied in 10 volunteers and it was found that tourniquet pain must have a significant cutaneous component since the tourniquet inflation time was tolerated longer with EMLA than with a placebo cream [7].

Clinical Experience

Testing of the EMLA cream has been carried out in many clinical applications. These included donor-site analgesia for split skin grafting; removal of molluscum contagiosum, tattoos and warts; and skin biopsies. The vast majority of clinical applications, however, has been for venous cannulation, especially in children. Pain associated with any punctures and fear of needles is a common problem associated with venous cannulation in children. Engberg and colleagues [4] tested the potential toxicity of EMLA in infants with regard to plasma concentration of prilocaine and lidocaine and also methemoglobin formation (ortotuloidine, a metabolite of prilocaine, is a methemoglobin-inducing agent). After application of 2 g of EMLA, i.e., 50 mg of lidocaine and 50 mg of prilocaine, on a 16 cm^2 area for 2–4 h in all cases the venous plasma concentrations of both drugs were found to be well below 200 ng/ml, which itself is far below toxic concentrations. The potential risk of methemoglobinemia was also ruled out. After an application time which was four times longer than the time required to produce analgesia, there was a slight but statistically significant increase in methemoglobin in the group of younger infants. The highest individual concentration found was 2%, which is still within the normal range. Their final recommendation was that EMLA could be used safely in infants older than 3 months.

In another investigation in older children (4–10 years) by Manner and colleagues [8], analgesia of the EMLA cream was demonstrated in a double blind randomized comparison between EMLA and a placebo cream. Median time of application and removal of the cream was approximately 1½ h. Pain assessment after insertion of iv cannula showed a marked analgesic effect, as expected from the EMLA group. Skin blanching was observed in both the EMLA and the placebo group in more than half the treated patients. On the other hand, venous determination of catecholamines and vasopressin, used in an attempt to quantitate stress due to anxiety, failed to demonstrate any significant difference between the EMLA group and the control group. Finally, the measured serum lidocaine concentrations after application of EMLA, in agreement with those reported by Engberg [4], were much lower than those connected with signs of toxicity. A similar study by Soliman et al. [10] compared EMLA with intradermal lidocaine infiltration prior to venous cannulation in unpremedicated children. The authors found that both methods were equally effective in producing analgesia but that the absence of pain did not necessarily improve a child's cooperation with venipuncture.

EMLA cream has also been widely tested in adults. One particular application has been in the treatment of postherpetic neuralgia, where both its pharmacodynamic and pharmacokinetic profile were studied [10]; 5% EMLA was applied for a 24 h period and was evaluated in 12 patients with refractory postherpetic neuralgia. The pain sensations were found to be significantly improved 6 h after application. Plasma concentrations of local anesthetics were also determined and found to be well below potentially toxic levels in all patients, even after such a prolonged application time. In another trial, EMLA was combined with glyceryl trinitrate in order not only to provide local anesthesia but also to vasodilate skin vessels in order to facilitate venipuncture [6]. Lower pain scores were found in both the EMLA group and the EMLA-glyceryl trinitrate group when compared to a placebo. Easier venipuncture was also found by the anesthesiologist when EMLA was used in combination with glyceryl trinitrate. In a double blind, double dummy study (four groups), the efficacy of 5% EMLA cream was assessed against that of lidocaine infiltration in pain relief during arterial cannulation. In this particularly well-designed study, significantly lower pain scores were observed by both patient and observer assessments in all patients receiving EMLA compared with those receiving placebo cream with lidocaine infiltration.

Conclusion

EMLA cream seems to be effective for percutaneous analgesia, especially for venipunctures both in children and in adults, where it seems to be more effective than infiltration of lidocaine. The prerequisites for the use of EMLA are an application under an occlusive dressing allowing a minimum of 60 min contact time with a careful site selection. Therefore, EMLA deserves a place in the routine armamentarium of premedication drugs for adults and children in selected cases.

References

1. Arendt-Nielsen L, Bjerring P (1988) Laser-induced pain for evaluation of local analgesia: A comparison of topical application (EMLA) and local injection (lidocaine). Anesth Analg 67: 115–123
2. Bjerring P, Andersen PH, Arendt-Nielsen L (1989) Vascular response of human skin after analgesia with EMLA cream. Br J Anaesth 63: 655–660
3. Bjerring P, Arendt-Nielsen L (1990) Depth and duration of skin analgesia to needle insertion after topical application of EMLA cream. Br DJ Anaesth 64: 173–177
4. Engberg G, Danielson K, Henneberg S, Nilsson A (1987) Plasma concentrations of prilocaine and lidocaine and methaemoglobin formation in infants after epicutaneous application of a 5% lidocaine-prilocaine cream (EMLA). Acta Anaesthesiol Scand 31: 624–628
5. Evers H, Von Dardel O, Juhlin L, Ohlsen L, Vinnars E (1985) Dermal effects of compositions based on the eutectic mixture of lignocaine and prilocaine (EMLA) – Studies in volunteers. Br J Anaesth 57: 997–1005
6. Gunawardene RD, Davenport HT (1990) Local application of EMLA and glyceryl trinitrate ointment before venipuncture. Anaesthesia 45: 52–54
7. Lowrie A, Jones MJ, Eastley RJ (1989) Effect of a eutectic mixture of local anaesthetic agents (EMLA) on tourniquet pain in volunteers. Br J Anaesth 63: 751–753
8. Manner T, Kanto J, Iisalo E, Lindgerg R, Viinamäki O, Scheinin M (1987) Reduction of pain at venous cannulation in children with a eutectic mixture of lidocaine and prilocaine (EMLA cream): Comparison with placebo cream and no local premedication. Acta Anaesthesiol Scand 31: 735–739
9. Smith M, Gray BM, Ingra S, Jewkes DA (1990) Double-blind comparison of topical lignocaine-prilocaine cream (EMLA) and lignocaine infiltration for arterial cannulation in adults. Br J Anaesth 65: 240–242
10. Soliman IE, Broadman LM, Hannallah RS, McGill WA (1988) Comparison of the analgesic effects of EMLA (Eutectic Mixture of Local Anesthetics) to intradermal lidocaine infiltration prior to venous cannulation in unpremedicated children. Anesthesiology 68: 804–806
11. Stow PJ, Glynn CJ, Minor B (1989) EMLA cream in the treatment of postherpetic neuralgia. Efficacy and pharmacokinetic profile. Pain 39:301–305

Scopolamine

I. TIGERSTEDT

Introduction

The incidence of nausea and vomiting in connection with anesthesia has not diminished, even with modern anesthesia techniques, since the 1930s when Waters reported an incidence of postoperative nausea and vomiting of about 40% [1].

In Finland, Janhunnen and Tammisto studied postoperative nausea after different types of general anesthesia in 1972 and found the incidence as high as 60% [3]. Later Korttila and coworkers (1979) reported an incidence of 55% after orthopedic surgery [5]. They studied several antiemetics: domperidone and metoclopramide (dopamine antagonists), and droperidol, a butyrophenone. They were able to demonstrate a significant reduction of postoperative nausea with droperidol (incidence only 25%). Since then we have used iv droperidol as our first choice postoperative antiemetic.

However, there are other groups of drugs currently used as antiemetics: antihistamines, phenothiazines, and anticholinergic drugs: atropine (hyoscyamine) and scopolamine (hyoscine).

Scopolamine TTS: Clinical Experience

Scopolamine was the first drug available as a transdermal preparation and was introduced in 1980 by Shaw and Urquhart [10]. Since scopolamine often causes drowsiness, blurred vision and even mental confusion in conventional parenteral form and dosage, the aim of the development program of transdermal scopolamine (TTS) was to minimize these effects and prolong the beneficial antiemetic effect. Shaw and Urquhart chose a drug entry of 5 μg/h into the blood to maintain the therapeutic antiemetic blood level for 72 h. A priming dose of 140 μg of scopolamine is first delivered from the transdermal preparation of which 100 μg binds to sites in the epidermis beneath the TTS adhesive with an area of 2.5 cm^2, and the remainder brings the blood levels to the steady-state concentration as soon as possible.

The TTS system has a multilayer construction comprising a steady-state reservoir in a gel form, a rate-controlling microporous membrane, and skin contact adhesive with the instant priming dose of scopolamine. This rate-controlled delivery system of a total dose of 0.5 mg produces its therapeutic antiemetic effect for 3 days with only about one-fifth of the dose required with a parenteral dosage (200 µg every 6 h for three days = 2.4 mg). The slow-release TTS patch should be applied to the retroauricular skin where the absortion is best and the delivery rate of the drug to the body depends on the formulation, and not on the nature of the skin [10].

We were interested to compare the efficacy of prophylactic transdermal scopolamine with droperidol since, in spite of reducing emetic symptoms, droperidol does not totally abolish postoperative sickness [5].

Ninety-six female patients scheduled for short-stay surgery (mainly on varicose veins) were randomly included in the study. The test drugs were given in a double blind, double dummy randomized manner. The patients were randomly allocated to three groups as follows:

TTS Group

Transdermal scopolamine, 0.5 mg/72 h (Scopoderm TTS, Ciba-Geigy), was used, delivering 140 µg scopolamine initially and thereafter 5 µg/h for up to 3 days. The scopolamine patch was placed retroauricularly in conjunction with im oxycodone premedication (0.13 mg/kg) about 1 h before the induction of anesthesia. The TTS patch was removed on the morning of the first postoperative day when the patients were discharged from hospital. Droperidol-placebo 0.5 ml was given iv 5 min before the end of surgery.

DHBP Group

Droperidol 1.25 mg (= 0.5 ml iv), was given 5 min before the end of surgery; A TTS-placebo patch was placed, as mentioned above.

Placebo Group

A Scopoderm-placebo patch and a DHBP-placebo, 0.5 ml iv, were administered, as mentioned above.

Anesthesia

Glycopyrrolate, 0.2 mg iv, was administered just prior to induction with thiopentone. Succinylcholine was given for endotracheal intubation and anesthesia was maintained with nitrous-oxide-oxygen, enflurane, fentanyl and vecuronium. At the end of surgery, muscular relaxation was antagonized iv with 0.4 mg glycopyrrolate and 2.0 mg neostigmine.

Results

The study groups were comparable in age, height, weight, duration of anesthesia, previous history of motion sickness, postoperative nausea and emesis during pregnancy. Also, the amounts of fentanyl given during anesthesia were similar (mean values 0.13–0.15 mg).

The incidence of nausea and vomiting was low and fairly similar in all study groups during the recovery room period of 2 h (Table 1). However, as a rescue medication, DHBP, 1.25 mg iv, was given more often to patients with TTS (28%) than to patients with DHBP (13%) or placebo (6%) and the difference between TTS and placebo groups was significant ($P < 0.05$) (Table 2). During the 24 postoperative hours on a surgical ward, fewer patients with TTS (63%) or DHBP (47%) experienced nausea than those with placebo (78%), the difference between DHBP and placebo being significant ($P < 0.05$). Vomiting was not significantly different in the three groups.

Side effects occured in all groups. Sedation was most frequent in the DHBP group and least frequent in the placebo. Dry mouth was complained of by

Table 1. Nausea and vomiting in the recovery room*

Recovery room	TTS	Placebo	DHBP
Nausea			
At arrival	8	3	5
At departure	2	3	1
Vomiting	9	3	5

* Number of patients: 32/group

Table 2. Antiemetic rescue medication (DHBP 1.25 iv) in the recovery room*

TTS	Placebo	DHBP
9**	2	4

* Number of patients: 32/group
** $P < 0.05$ compared to placebo

Table 3. Nausea and vomiting on the ward (in the first 24 h postoperatively)

	TTS	Placebo	DHBP
Nausea	20	25	15**
Vomiting	13	19	12

* Number of patients: 32/group
** $P < 0.05$ compared to placebo

Table 4. Side effects in the recovery room

	TTS	Placebo	DHBP
Sedation			
At arrival	12	6	21*
At departure	10	5	9
Dry mouth	20	20	18
Blurred vision	12*	2	2

* $P < 0.01$ compared to placebo

18–20 patients in each group. Blurred vision was significantly more frequent after TTS ($P < 0.01$).

Discussion

We realized that TTS with intramuscular oxycodone premedication did not significantly reduce the overall incidence of postoperative emetic sequelae. As a consequence we are not using TTS as a first choice antiemetic for postoperative nausea.

Earlier investigators have reported better results for TTS. According to Uppington [12], a reduction from 100% to 68% could be achieved with TTS during the first 24 h after major gynecological surgery. After similar surgery, Tolksdorf [11] observed a reduction from 75% to 45%. Treating children after eye surgery, Gibbons [2] did not find any significant reduction of nausea with the use of TTS but one-fifth of the children experienced anxiety and hallucinations. Waldvogel found an incidence of 47% of nausea while using TTS after various surgical procedures [13]. According to Loper et al. [7] TTS also reduced nausea in patients with epidural morphine after gynecological surgery.

In Finland, however, a recent study by Koski and coworkers [6] showed no difference in nausea and vomiting between TTS and placebo after balanced

Table 5. Postoperative antiemetic studies. Nausea and vomiting after:

	TTS (%)	Placebo (%)	DHBP (%)
Waldvogel [13]	47	—	20
Gibbons et al. [2]	26	38	—
Tolksdorf et al. [11]	45	75	—
Uppington et al. [12]	68	100	—
Korttila et al. [5]	—	55	25
Tigerstedt et al. (1988)	63	78	47
Koski et al. [6]	54	57	—

anesthesia for gynecological surgery. In their study, TTS was applied on the evening before surgery, as recommended by the manufacturer for better steady-state concentration during anesthesia with enflurane and fentanyl supplementation. Earlier administration did not, however, improve the results with TTS. It therefore seems that the true value of TTS as a postoperative antiemetic is still unsettled.

Postoperative nausea and vomiting are rarely the result of one factor [9] and therefore its treatment can often be difficult. Anticholinergic drugs are probably the most widely used antiemetics. Though TTS has been shown to prevent seasickness in several studies, the CNS mechanism of seasickness is different from that of postoperative emesis. In seasickness the stimuli arise from the vestibular organ, causing an imbalance between the cholinergic and noradrenergic systems of the vomiting center. Postoperative nausea is mainly due to drugs acting on the dopaminergic receptor sites of the chemoreceptor trigger zone, from where impulses are relayed to the closely associated vomiting center [8].

The activity of anticholinergics such as scopolamine and atropine (but not glycopyrrolate) at the muscarinic cholinergic neurotransmitter receptor sites is different from that of droperidol, which is a strong antidopaminergic agent. This difference may explain the inferior effect of scopolamine on postoperative nausea.

References

1. Editorial (1986) Transdermal hyoscine (scopolamine) and postoperative vomiting. Anaesthesia 41: 1–3
2. Gibbons PA, Nicolson SC, Betts EK, Rosenberry KR, Jobes DR (1984) Scopolamine does not not prevent postoperative emesis after pediatric eye surgery. Anesthesiology 61: A435
3. Janhunen L, Tammisto T (1972) Postoperative vomiting after different types of general anaesthesia. Ann Chir Gynaecol Fenn 61: 152–159
4. Kauste A, Tuominen M, Heikkinen H, Gordin A, Korttila K (1986) Droperidol, alitsapride and metoclopramide in the prevention and treatment of postoperative emetic sequelae. Eur J Anaesth 3: 1–9
5. Korttila K, Kauste A, Auvinen J (1979) Comparison of domperidone, droperidol and metoclopramide in the prevention and treatment of nausea and vomiting after balanced general anaesthesia. Anesth Analg 58: 396–400
6. Koski EMJ, Mattila MAK, Knapik D, Toivanen T, Ruusukallio H, Andersson P, Freudenthal Y (1990) Double blind comparison of transdermal hyoscine and placebo for the prevention of postoperative nausea. Br J Anaesth 64: 16–20
7. Loper KA, Ready B, Dorman BH (1989) Prophylactic transdermal scopolamine patches reduce nausea in postoperative patients receiving epidural morphine. Anesth Analg 68: 144–146
8. Palazzo MGA, Strunin L (1984a) Anaesthesia and Emesis I. Etiology. Can Anaesth Soc J 31: 178–187
9. Palazzo MGA, Strunin L (1984b) Anaesthesia and Emesis II: Prevention and management. Can Anaesth Soc J 31: 407–415
10. Shaw J, Urquhart J (1980) Programmed, systemic drug delivery by the transdermal route. Trends Pharmacol Sci 1: 208–211

11. Tolksdorf W, Meisel R, Müller P, Bender H-J (1985) Transdermales Scopolamin (TTS-Scopolamin) zur Prophylaxe postoperativer Übelkeit und Erbrechen. Anaesthesist 34: 656–662
12. Uppington J, Dunnet J, Blogg CE (1986) Transdermal hyoscine and postoperative nausea and vomiting. Anaesthesia 41: 16–20
13. Waldvogel HH (1983) Transdermales Scopolamin gegen postoperatives Erbrechen: Eine neue Prämedikationsformel? Anästh Intensivther Notfallmed 18: 258–2607

Subject Index

GPSR Compliance

The European Union's (EU) General Product Safety Regulation (GPSR) is a set of rules that requires consumer products to be safe and our obligations to ensure this.

If you have any concerns about our products, you can contact us on ProductSafety@springernature.com

In case Publisher is established outside the EU, the EU authorized representative is:

Springer Nature Customer Service Center GmbH
Europaplatz 3
69115 Heidelberg, Germany

Batch number: 10583998

Printed by Printforce, the Netherlands